PHYSICAL DIAGNOSIS

MEDICAL EXAMINATION REVIEW

PHYSICAL DIAGNOSIS

Third Edition

550 Multiple-Choice Questions
with Referenced, Explanatory Answers

John H. Holbrook, M.D., F.A.C.P.
Associate Professor of Internal Medicine
University of Utah School of Medicine
Salt Lake City, Utah

MEDICAL EXAMINATION PUBLISHING COMPANY

NOTICE

The authors and publisher of this book have made every effort to ensure that all therapeutic modalities that are recommended are in accordance with accepted standards at the time of publication.

The drugs specified within this book may not have specific approval by the Food and Drug Administration in regard to the indications and dosages that are recommended by the authors. The manufacturer's package insert is the best source of current prescribing information.

Medical Examination Publishing Company
A Division of Elsevier Science Publishing Co., Inc.
52 Vanderbilt Avenue, New York, New York 10017

Library of Congress Cataloging in Publication Data

The Library of Congress has cataloged the set as follows:

Medical examination review.—Flushing, N.Y.: Medical Examination Pub. Co.,
1960–<1981 >
v. <1–9, 12–32, 34–37 >: ill. ; 22cm.
Vol. published in Garden City, N.Y.
Includes various editions of some volumes.
Published 1960–1980 as: Medical examination review book.
Includes bibliographical references.
LC holdings recorded in Shelflist only as of 6/25/81.

1. Medicine—Examinations, questions, etc.
RC58.M4 610'.76—dc19 61-66847
ISBN 0-444-01122-6 AACR 2 MARC

Current printing (last digit):
10 9 8 7 6 5 4 3 2 1

Manufactured in the United States of America

Contents

Preface

Modern medicine tends to underestimate the importance of clinical skills. This is unfortunate because the history and physical examination usually provide a cost-effective, safe framework for the appropriate use of the laboratory. Furthermore, the bedside examination continues to provide essential data that may not be obtainable from laboratory studies.

This book was written to encourage the development and improvement of clinical skills. The expert clinician is a permanent student who expands and refines bedside skills through examining patients, consulting with colleagues, and regularly studying medical literature. Inexperienced clinicians will benefit by assessing their understanding of fundamental concepts and techniques. Accomplished clinicians may discover overlooked "pearls" and recently published studies.

Emphasis is placed on physiologic and pathophysiologic mechanisms, interpretation of data, and methods of examination. Explanatory answers are included to facilitate selective in-depth study through reference to standard textbooks and selected journal articles.

The author is indebted to his colleagues at the University of Utah School of Medicine for their helpful comments, to his wife, Judith M. Holbrook, for her support and encouragement, and to Mary Lou Benson for her assistance in preparing the manuscript.

Disclaimer

The author has made every effort to verify thoroughly the answers to the questions that appear on the following pages. However, as in any text, some inaccuracies and ambiguities may occur; therefore, if in doubt, please consult your references.

The Publisher

1 The Abdomen

DIRECTIONS: Each of the questions or incomplete statements below is followed by five suggested answers or completions. Select the **one** that is best in each case.

---

1. Select the INCORRECT statement concerning the technique of abdominal palpation.

A. The patient should be in the supine position with the knees flexed
B. The examiner should stand on the patient's right side
C. The patient's abdomen should be exposed from the diaphragm to the groin
D. The examiner's hand should be maintained in a plane parallel to the bed
E. Palpation for the liver edge should begin in the right upper quadrant

2. Which of the following structures is abnormal when it is palpable?

A. Colon
B. Liver
C. Kidney
D. Spleen
E. Aorta

3. In a study of patients with possible ascites the sensitivity and specificity of several physical signs were compared. Ultrasonography was utilized as a reference standard. Select the sign with the highest sensitivity.
A. Bulging flanks
B. Flank dullness
C. Shifting dullness
D. A fluid wave
E. A positive "puddle" sign

4. A sign that confirms the presence of peritonitis is
A. ileus
B. borborygmus
C. rebound tenderness
D. voluntary abdominal wall rigidity
E. direct tenderness

5. Slight jaundice is often first noted by examining the
A. urine
B. stool
C. skin
D. sclera
E. nails

6. The earliest clinical recognition of jaundice is usually correlated with a total serum bilirubin of at least
A. 1.0 mg%
B. 2.0 mg%
C. 3.0 mg%
D. 4.0 mg%
E. 5.0 mg%

7. A femoral hernia
A. lies medial to the pubic tubercle
B. lies below the inguinal ligament
C. does not reduce
D. is not associated with an impulse on coughing
E. passes through Hesselbach's triangle

8. A focus of purulent drainage located in the sacrococcygeal area cephalad to the anus, in the midline, is noted to contain tufts of hair. This is most likely

A. a sebaceous cyst
B. an anal fissure
C. an anorectal fistula
D. a pilonidal cyst
E. an ischiorectal abscess

9. In a patient with tense ascites, hepatosplenomegaly may be best detected by

A. the hooking maneuver
B. percussion
C. palpation
D. ballottement
E. observation with deep respiration

10. In the presence of biliary colic the patient usually

A. moves restlessly
B. lies quietly in the supine position
C. lies with his knees drawn up
D. lies on his right side
E. lies with his right thigh flexed

11. In order to document absent bowel sounds, the examiner should carefully auscultate for at least

A. 30 seconds
B. 1 minute
C. 2 minutes
D. 3 minutes
E. 5 minutes

12. Which of the following is an almost constant finding with a perforated peptic ulcer?

A. Fever
B. Shifting dullness
C. Rigidity of the abdominal wall
D. Shoulder pain
E. Lightheadedness

13. The initial pain of appendicitis is usually referred
A. to the epigastric or periumbilical area
B. diffusely to the right lower quadrant
C. to McBurney's point
D. to the right flank
E. to the entire abdomen

14. A 45-year-old woman with acute upper abdominal pain is asked to inspire as an examiner's fingers are inserted deeply under the right costal margin. The patient suddenly stops inspiring because of sharp pain. The most likely diagnosis is
A. acute gastroenteritis
B. acute cholecystitis
C. a duodenal ulcer
D. acute pancreatitis
E. acute pyelonephritis

15. The correct sequence of signs and symptoms seen with acute appendicitis is
A. epigastric pain, nausea or vomiting, local iliac tenderness, fever
B. nausea or vomiting, epigastric pain, local iliac tenderness, fever
C. fever, epigastric pain, nausea or vomiting, local iliac tenderness
D. local iliac tenderness, epigastric pain, nausea or vomiting, fever
E. epigastric pain, fever, nausea or vomiting, local iliac tenderness

16. McBurney's point lies
A. at the midpoint of a line connecting the right midinguinal ligament and the umbilicus
B. at the midpoint of a line connecting the right pubic tubercle and the umbilicus
C. at the midpoint of a line connecting the right anterior superior iliac spine and the umbilicus
D. 2 in. from the right anterior superior iliac spine on a line connecting the umbilicus and the spine
E. 2 in. from the right midinguinal ligament on a line connecting the umbilicus and the ligament

17. A patient's liver is noted to be pulsatile. The most likely explanation for this is
A. portal hypertension
B. severe tricuspid insufficiency
C. aortic insufficiency
D. a hepatoma
E. tricuspid stenosis

18. On digital rectal examination of a 50-year-old man, a bilobed, 3 × 4-cm structure is palpated anteriorly. It is firm and projects 2–3 mm into the rectal lumen. This is most likely
A. an internal hemorrhoid
B. a normal prostate gland
C. a prostatic carcinoma
D. a rectal polyp
E. prostatic hypertrophy

19. When examining the abdomen, which one of the following procedures should immediately follow inspection?
A. Percussion
B. Palpation
C. A rectal examination
D. Auscultation
E. Ballottement

20. As a supine patient elevates his head, a midline abdominal ridge appears, which extends from the xiphoid to the pubic crest. The most likely diagnosis is
A. meteorism
B. a spigelian hernia
C. an umbilical hernia
D. a linea alba hernia
E. a diastasis recti

21. The diagnosis of internal hemorrhoids is established by
A. inspection
B. digital rectal examination
C. anoscopy
D. the history
E. the stool guaiac test

22. Epigastric abdominal bruits are most commonly due to narrowing of which artery?
A. Celiac artery
B. Superior mesenteric artery
C. Renal artery
D. Aorta
E. Splenic artery

23. A patient notes "heartburn" especially when lying down. This is most likely due to
A. acute cholecystitis
B. reflux esophagitis
C. a duodenal ulcer
D. pancreatitis
E. coronary artery disease

24. A continuous venous hum heard over the abdomen strongly suggests the diagnosis of
A. portal hypertension
B. metastatic carcinoma
C. the Budd–Chiari syndrome
D. splenomegaly
E. an aortic aneurysm

25. A patient's hernia involves only part of the bowel circumference. Which type of hernia is this?
A. Spigelian
B. Ventral
C. Richter
D. Littre
E. Umbilical

26. A patient demonstrates distended anterior abdominal wall veins. The upper abdominal veins drain downward. This observation
A. suggests the diagnosis of portal hypertension
B. is normal
C. suggests the diagnosis of superior vena caval obstruction
D. suggests the diagnosis of inferior vena caval obstruction
E. is clinically insignificant

27. Digital rectal examination can be expected to detect approximately what percent of rectal cancers?
A. 10%
B. 20%
C. 30%
D. 40%
E. 50%

28. Anterior abdominal wall pulsations, which correspond to the cardiac cycle, are noted below the umbilicus. This suggests the diagnosis of
A. a normal transmitted pulsation
B. coarctation of the aorta
C. an aortic aneurysm
D. a thin anterior abdominal wall
E. the hyperkinetic cardiac syndrome

29. A 54-year-old man presents in an emergency room with diffuse abdominal pain, hypotension, and flank ecchymoses. The most likely diagnosis is
A. cholecystitis
B. esophagitis
C. retroperitoneal hemorrhage
D. renal colic
E. peritonitis

30. All of the following structures lie in the transpyloric plane EXCEPT the
A. renal artery
B. first part of the duodenum
C. pancreas
D. adrenal gland
E. transverse colon

31. A patient develops an acute bowel obstruction. Auscultation of the abdomen would be expected to demonstrate
A. borborygmi
B. absent bowel sounds
C. decreased bowel sounds
D. slightly increased bowel sounds
E. normal bowel sounds

DIRECTIONS: Each of the questions or incomplete statements below is followed by five suggested answers or completions. Select either true (T) or false (F) for **each** option given.

32. Splenomegaly is commonly associated with
A. sickle-cell anemia
B. thalassemia major
C. chronic myelocytic leukemia
D. Felty's syndrome
E. myelofibrosis

33. Unilateral costovertebral angle tenderness suggests the diagnosis of
A. cholecystitis
B. a perinephric abscess
C. cystitis
D. pancreatitis
E. pyelonephritis

34. Visible peristalsis may be seen
A. in thin, normal individuals
B. with ascites
C. with peritonitis
D. with subacute intestinal obstruction
E. with constipation

35. Liver height determined by percussion in the midclavicular line
A. correlates well with liver scan results
B. is independent of percussion technique
C. tends to be larger in males than females
D. should be less than 12 cm in normal adults
E. is independent of lean body mass

36. A 50-year-old man's liver is palpable 5 cm below the right costal margin. The vertical liver span is 10 cm. Conditions that might be associated with these findings include

A. polycystic liver disease
B. a right-sided pleural effusion
C. chronic obstructive pulmonary disease
D. a hepatoma
E. ptosis of the liver

37. Visceral pain referred to the epigastrium may originate from the

A. stomach
B. duodenum
C. gallbladder
D. pancreas
E. colon

38. A rectal examination in a patient with an uncomplicated acute myocardial infarction

A. is hazardous and should not be done
B. may be safely done
C. often provokes arrhythmias
D. often precipitates angina pectoris
E. provides important data concerning patient management

2 The Breast

DIRECTIONS: Each of the questions or incomplete statements below is followed by five suggested answers or completions. Select the **one** that is best in each case.

39. Carcinoma of the breast is found most frequently in the
A. upper outer quadrant
B. subareolar area
C. upper inner quadrant
D. lower outer quadrant
E. lower inner quadrant

40. A female patient with a chronic eczematous lesion of the nipple should be studied to exclude the diagnosis of
A. chronic cystic mastitis
B. atopic dermatitis
C. Paget's disease
D. traumatic fat necrosis
E. a fibroadenoma

41. A bloody nipple discharge is usually due to
A. a breast carcinoma
B. chronic cystic mastitis
C. a benign intraductal papilloma
D. Paget's disease
E. a fibroadenoma

42. Carcinoma of the male breast is usually found
A. in the upper outer quadrant
B. in the upper inner quadrant
C. beneath the nipple or areola
D. in the lower inner quadrant
E. in the lower outer quadrant

43. "Retraction phenomena" of the breast are due to
A. blockage of lymphatics
B. direct fixation of abnormal tissue to the chest wall
C. atrophy
D. increased capillary permeability
E. fibrotic changes in the suspensory ligaments

44. Gynecomastia is usually diagnosed by
A. observation
B. palpation
C. mammography
D. biopsy
E. thermography

45. An afebrile, nonlactating woman develops acute inflammation of the breast. She should be examined for
A. duct ectasia
B. lymphangitis
C. infectious mastitis
D. a breast abscess
E. an inflammatory breast carcinoma

46. Breast examination of a 40-year-old woman reveals multiple tender nodules. She recalls that the tenderness is intermittent, and that the nodules have appeared over a period of years. The most likely diagnosis is
A. a breast carcinoma
B. chronic cystic mastitis
C. fibroadenomas
D. lipomas
E. a normal variant

47. Asymptomatic gynecomastia
A. suggests the diagnosis of breast cancer
B. is a common finding in normal patients
C. is rarely related to drug use
D. should be routinely biopsied
E. is unusual in teenage boys

48. The most sensitive screening tool for breast cancer is
A. thermography
B. the physical examination
C. mammography
D. self-examination
E. the physical examination and mammography

49. A 30-year-old woman notes a nontender, well-defined breast "lump." The most likely diagnosis is
A. a carcinoma
B. a chronic abscess
C. a sarcoma
D. a fibroadenoma
E. fat necrosis

DIRECTIONS: Each of the questions or incomplete statements below is followed by five suggested answers or completions. Select either true (T) or false (F) for **each** option given.

---

50. Palpatory features of a breast "lump" that suggest a carcinoma include it
A. is freely movable
B. is tender on palpation
C. has irregular margins
D. is a single dominant mass
E. is hard

51. Which of the following are normal anatomical variants of the breast?

A. The inframammary fold
B. Unilateral venous prominence
C. The axillary tail of the breast
D. Chronic nipple inversion
E. Areolar edema

52. Which of the following may produce a hard, poorly defined breast mass with skin retraction?

A. A carcinoma
B. Duct ectasia
C. Traumatic fat necrosis
D. A fibroadenoma
E. A low-grade abscess

3 The Chest and Lungs

DIRECTIONS: Each of the questions or incomplete statements below is followed by five suggested answers or completions. Select the **one** that is best in each case.

53. The normal breath sounds heard over most of the lung fields are
A. bronchial
B. bronchovesicular
C. vesicular
D. tracheal
E. bronchotracheal

54. A patient without underlying lung disease develops a right pleural effusion. All of the following might be present on the right side EXCEPT
A. dullness to percussion
B. diminished breath sounds
C. decreased tactile fremitus
D. egophony
E. rales

55. All of the following physical findings are expected in a patient with pneumonia except
A. increased fremitus
B. dullness to percussion
C. vesicular breath sounds
D. bronchophony
E. pectoriloquy

56. Vocal fremitus should be increased with
- **A.** obesity
- **B.** a pneumothorax
- **C.** a pleural effusion
- **D.** pneumonia
- **E.** a thickened pleura

57. In a patient with emphysema the heart sounds may be heard best
- **A.** in the epigastrium
- **B.** at the apex
- **C.** at the right second interspace
- **D.** at the left second interspace
- **E.** at the left fourth interspace

58. All of the following physical findings are anticipated with a pneumothorax EXCEPT
- **A.** absent tactile fremitus
- **B.** reduced chest expansion on inspiration
- **C.** decreased resonance to percussion on the involved side
- **D.** deviation of the trachea to the involved side
- **E.** reduced breath sounds

59. Rales are probably produced by
- **A.** turbulent air flow
- **B.** the opening of previously closed small airways
- **C.** laminar airflow
- **D.** airway obstruction
- **E.** none of the above

60. Which is the feature of a pleural friction rub that is LEAST helpful in distinguishing it from a rhonchus?
- **A.** A pleural rub is unaffected by coughing
- **B.** A pleural rub has a grating quality
- **C.** A pleural rub sounds close to the ear
- **D.** A pleural rub is usually heard on inspiration and expiration
- **E.** A pleural rub is amplified by pressing on the stethoscope

61. Because of the lungs' anatomy, the physical findings of pneumonia may be confined to a very localized area. This is especially true when pneumonia involves the
A. right upper lobe
B. right middle lobe
C. right lower lobe
D. left upper lobe
E. left lower lobe

62. A stridor indicates
A. bronchostenosis
B. a tension pneumothorax
C. upper airway obstruction
D. asthma
E. severe emphysema

63. The most useful distinguishing characteristic of the different types of breath sounds is
A. location
B. pitch
C. quality
D. intensity
E. relative duration of inspiration and expiration

64. When examining the lung fields, posteriorly, it is important to recognize that the lower lobes extend up to the level of
A. C-7
B. T-2
C. T-4
D. T-6
E. T-8

65. Respiratory excursion is appreciated best when the hands are placed
A. at the posterior lung bases
B. over the apices
C. along the horizontal fissure of the midaxillary line
D. over the scapulas
E. along the lower anterolateral chest wall

66. The basic pathophysiologic process accounting for retraction of the intercostal spaces is

A. decreased pulmonary compliance
B. inspiratory airway obstruction
C. expiratory airway obstruction
D. pulmonary hypertension
E. pulmonary fibrosis

67. Normally, after deep inhalation, a patient should be able to forcibly expire the air from the lungs in

A. 2.5 seconds or less
B. 3.0 seconds or less
C. 3.5 seconds or less
D. 4.0 seconds or less
E. 4.5 seconds or less

68. The normal inspiratory/expiratory time ratio with quiet breathing is

A. 3:1
B. 2:1
C. 1:1
D. 1:2
E. 1:3

69. According to studies using time-expanded wave-form analysis, the most correct descriptive phrase concerning a rale is

A. a discontinuous sound
B. a continuous sound
C. an inspiratory sound
D. an expiratory sound
E. both an inspiratory and expiratory sound

70. The characteristic physical finding of bronchial asthma is the

A. wheeze
B. rub
C. crackle
D. stridor
E. rale

71. An "A" sound is heard while auscultating over the lung fields as the patient says "E." This is
   A. vocal fremitus
   B. egophony
   C. pectoriloquy
   D. a wheeze
   E. bronchial breathing

72. Breathing through pursed lips suggests the diagnosis of
   A. pulmonary hypertension
   B. primary hypoventilation
   C. tracheal obstruction
   D. emphysema
   E. interstitial fibrosis

73. The normal percussion note heard over most of the lung during most of the respiratory cycle is
   A. tympany
   B. resonance
   C. hyperresonance
   D. dullness
   E. flatness

74. The most effective tool for comparing the state of bronchial patency in different parts of the bronchopulmonary tree is
   A. a chest film
   B. percussion
   C. observation
   D. palpation
   E. auscultation

75. After shallow breathing, auscultation may normally reveal
   A. egophony
   B. a few basilar end-inspiratory rales
   C. pectoriloquy
   D. wheezes
   E. bronchophony

76. Low, fixed diaphragms are characteristic of
- **A.** severe emphysema
- **B.** chronic bronchitis
- **C.** congestive heart failure
- **D.** bronchiectasis
- **E.** interstitial fibrosis

77. Auscultatory percussion appears to be a sensitive technique for detecting all of the following EXCEPT
- **A.** pneumonia
- **B.** emphysema
- **C.** lung cancer
- **D.** benign lung masses
- **E.** tuberculosis

78. The recommended new American Thoracic Society term for "rale" is
- **A.** crackle
- **B.** wheeze
- **C.** rhonchus
- **D.** rub
- **E.** crepitation

79. A fixed, monophonic wheeze is characteristically produced by all of the following EXCEPT
- **A.** asthma
- **B.** a tumor
- **C.** a granuloma
- **D.** a foreign body
- **E.** bronchial scarring with stenosis

80. Current evidence suggests that normal vesicular breath sounds arise in the
- **A.** alveolus
- **B.** alveolar duct
- **C.** respiratory bronchiole
- **D.** terminal bronchiole
- **E.** bronchus

81. A continuous chest bruit is heard in a patient with shortness of breath. At the point where the bruit is heard best, a chest film demonstrates a rounded mass. The physical finding that would strongly suggest the underlying diagnosis is
A. telangiectasia
B. lymphadenopathy
C. hepatomegaly
D. cardiomegaly
E. clubbing

82. Active abdominal contraction with each respiratory cycle
A. is a normal variant
B. suggests an anxiety reaction
C. suggests inspiratory airway obstruction
D. suggests expiratory airway obstruction
E. suggests a flail chest

83. Apical posttussive rales are most likely due to
A. asthma
B. chronic bronchitis
C. congestive heart failure
D. tuberculosis
E. interstitial pulmonary fibrosis

84. A 70-year-old man with severe kyphoscoliosis is admitted to the hospital with heart failure. Cardiopulmonary evaluation will probably demonstrate all of the following EXCEPT
A. increased airway resistance
B. reduction in lung volume
C. hypoxemia
D. ventilation/perfusion mismatching
E. pulmonary hypertension

85. All of the following disorders are associated with crackles that occur characteristically in late inspiration EXCEPT
A. sarcoidosis
B. asbestosis
C. severe emphysema
D. interstitial fibrosis
E. scleroderma lung disease

DIRECTIONS: Each of the questions or incomplete statements below is followed by five suggested answers or completions. Select either true (T) or false (F) for **each** option given.

86. Features of rhonchi that distinguish them from rales include
- **A.** they are usually present during both inspiration and expiration
- **B.** they consist of a series of discontinuous sounds
- **C.** they are often more prominent during expiration than inspiration
- **D.** they are produced by airway narrowing
- **E.** they are produced by opening of hypoventilated areas

87. Labored respiration is suggested by
- **A.** a respiratory rate of 20 breaths/min
- **B.** diaphragmatic breathing in a male
- **C.** intercostal retractions
- **D.** an excessively long expiratory phase
- **E.** use of the accessory muscles of respiration

88. Bronchial breath sounds
- **A.** are low-pitched
- **B.** have a longer expiratory phase than vesicular breath sounds
- **C.** are abnormal if heard over the chest except over the manubrium
- **D.** are produced by alveolar distention
- **E.** are usually louder than vesicular breath sounds

89. A unilateral decrease in chest expansion may be seen
- **A.** as a normal variant
- **B.** with a rib fracture
- **C.** with a pleural effusion
- **D.** with a phrenic nerve palsy
- **E.** with pneumonia

90. Vocal fremitus
- **A.** differs from tactile fremitus
- **B.** is more readily perceived with a low-pitched voice
- **C.** is normally most intense at the lung bases
- **D.** is significantly increased with pneumonia
- **E.** is due to the transmission of laryngeal vibrations to the chest wall

91. Which of the following are correct statements concerning the surface anatomy of the chest?
- **A.** The bifurcation of the trachea lies at the suprasternal notch
- **B.** The scapulae lie approximately between the second and eighth ribs
- **C.** The first rib articulates with the angle of Louis
- **D.** The most readily identifiable cervical vertebra is C-7
- **E.** The apices of the lungs extend approximately 3 cm above the clavicles

4 The Ears, Nose, and Throat

DIRECTIONS: Each of the questions or incomplete statements below is followed by five suggested answers or completions. Select the **one** that is best in each case.

---

92. Correct steps for otoscopic examination of the adult include all of the following EXCEPT

A. inspect the external canal before introducing the speculum

B. choose the largest speculum that can be introduced into the canal without causing pain

C. straighten the external canal by pulling the pinna horizontally backwards

D. guard against sudden patient movement that might result in trauma to the external canal

E. adjust the line of vision to allow observation of the entire canal and tympanic membrane

93. Exacerbation of ear pain upon moving the auricle suggests the diagnosis of

A. otitis media

B. mastoiditis

C. impacted cerumen

D. parotitis

E. otitis externa

94. A progressive nonfluctuating unilateral hearing loss, unilateral tinnitus, and unsteadiness suggest the diagnosis of
- **A.** Meniere's disease
- **B.** an acoustic neuroma
- **C.** presbycusis
- **D.** otosclerosis
- **E.** hereditary deafness

95. A chronic asthmatic is noted to have nasal polyps. The patient should avoid all of the following EXCEPT
- **A.** aspirin
- **B.** indomethacin
- **C.** sodium salicylate
- **D.** mephenamic acid
- **E.** tartrazine yellow

96. Which is the tuning fork of choice for performing the Weber test?
- **A.** 128 cycles/sec
- **B.** 256 cycles/sec
- **C.** 512 cycles/sec.
- **D.** 1024 cycles/sec.
- **E.** 2048 cycles/sec.

97. Bluish-tinted ears and black-colored cerumen suggest the diagnosis of
- **A.** cyanosis
- **B.** osteogenesis imperfecta
- **C.** a melanoma
- **D.** ochronosis
- **E.** Addison's disease

98. A retracted tympanic membrane is produced by
- **A.** eustachian tube obstruction
- **B.** otitis externa
- **C.** purulent otitis media
- **D.** mastoiditis
- **E.** myringitis

99. A 16-year-old girl develops a painful ear, sore throat, cough, and fever. Physical examination reveals an inflamed pharynx and inflamed tympanic membranes with hemorrhagic vesicles. The most likely diagnosis is
A. otitis externa
B. a pneumococcal infection
C. a streptococcal infection
D. a mycoplasma infection
E. serous otitis media

100. A "hairy" tongue is due to
A. proliferation of fungiform papillae
B. lengthening of filiform papillae
C. hirsutism
D. fissuring of the dorsal surface of the tongue
E. hypertrophy of the circumvallate papillae

101. A very hard protuberance in the midline of the hard palate is probably
A. leukoplakia
B. enlarged adenoids
C. a torus palatinus
D. a hyperplastic response to dentures
E. a palatine carcinoma

102. A chronic, white, indurated oral mucosal lesion is noted. A premalignant disorder that must be excluded is
A. leukoplakia
B. candidiasis
C. lichen planus
D. pachyderma oris
E. aphthous stomatitis

103. A patient's tongue demonstrates asymptomatic migratory red patches. This is
A. a "strawberry" tongue
B. an atrophic tongue
C. a "scrotal" tongue
D. a "geographic" tongue
E. a coated tongue

104. A patient with putrid breath should be suspected of having
A. diabetic ketoacidosis
B. uremia
C. an anaerobic lung infection
D. fetor hepaticus
E. alcoholic intoxication

105. A 14-year-old teenager's gums are noted to be hypertrophied. All of the following may account for this problem EXCEPT
A. penicillin therapy
B. pregnancy
C. puberty
D. leukemia
E. diphenylhydantoin therapy

106. When examining the mouth, it is important to remember that the most common site of oral cancer is the
A. tongue
B. palate
C. lip
D. buccal mucosa
E. sublingual space

107. The most specific finding to support the diagnosis of acute sinusitis is
A. a purulent nasal discharge
B. boggy nasal mucosa
C. asymmetrical sinus transillumination
D. purulent drainage from a sinus ostium
E. focal sinus tenderness

108. Maxillary sinus tenderness and swelling are most likely due to
A. vasomotor rhinitis
B. a dental abscess
C. maxillary sinusitis
D. a maxillary carcinoma
E. an antral cyst

109. The reliable detection of serous otitis depends upon
A. recognizing a retracted tympanic membrane
B. noting a slate-gray color of the tympanic membrane
C. checking for tympanic membrane mobility with the pneumatic otoscope
D. observing air bubbles behind the tympanic membrane
E. observing a fluid level

110. The most likely cause for brownish mottling and pitting of a patient's teeth is
A. maternal ingestion of tetracycline during pregnancy
B. erythroblastosis fetalis
C. congenital syphilis
D. congenital rubella
E. fluorosis

111. Multiple, pinhead-sized, yellow macules are present on the buccal mucosa, bilaterally. They are asymptomatic. The most likely diagnosis is
A. leukoplakia
B. Koplik's spots
C. sebaceous glands
D. retention cysts
E. oral moniliasis

112. A slowly progressive, bulbous nasal deformity is due to
A. a basal cell carcinoma
B. relapsing polychondritis
C. acne rosacea
D. actinic keratosis
E. systemic lupus erythematosus

113. Hard, white deposits found along the helix of the ear suggest the diagnosis of
A. chondrocalcinosis
B. relapsing polychondritis
C. gout
D. a squamous cell carcinoma
E. Darwin's tubercle

114. A patient with enlarged, orange tonsils should be evaluated for
A. a lymphoma
B. type III hyperlipoproteinemia
C. hypercarotinemia
D. Tangier disease
E. primary biliary cirrhosis

115. A 26-year-old man develops a severe sore throat and fever. Examination demonstrates hoarseness, a stridor, and drooling. The most likely diagnosis is
A. diphtheria
B. acute laryngitis
C. acute pharyngitis
D. acute epiglottitis
E. a retropharyngeal abscess

116. A 30-year-old, white, male patient presents in an emergency room with fever, diffuse lymphadenopathy, and 2 × 3-cm areas of raised, white plaques on the lateral margins of the tongue. The lesions do not rub off and feature numerous projections. The most likely diagnosis is
A. a geographic tongue
B. leukoplakia
C. glossitis
D. thrush
E. "hairy" leukoplakia

117. The color of the normal tympanic membrane is
A. pink
B. pearly gray
C. blue
D. white
E. red

118. Otoscopic examination of the tympanic membrane reveals a white, nodular lesion near the periphery. The most likely diagnosis is
- **A.** a carcinoma
- **B.** an osteoma
- **C.** a cholesteatoma
- **D.** chronic otitis externa
- **E.** a carotid body tumor

119. A 26-year-old man has had recurrent episodes of epistaxis. Physical examination reveals numerous telangiectasia on the lips, tongue, and palms. The most likely diagnosis is
- **A.** trauma
- **B.** a coagulopathy
- **C.** a nasal infection
- **D.** hereditary hemorrhagic telangiectasia
- **E.** hypertension

DIRECTIONS: Each of the questions or incomplete statements below is followed by five suggested answers or completions. Select either true (T) or false (F) for **each** option given.

---

120. True statements concerning the use of the tuning fork for evaluation of auditory acuity include
- **A.** a positive Rinne test is normal
- **B.** the use of the tuning fork is outmoded
- **C.** air conduction is normally greater than bone conduction
- **D.** the Weber test measures air conduction
- **E.** the Weber test lateralizes to the side of a conductive loss because environmental noise is masked

121. A smooth, beefy-appearing tongue may be due to
- **A.** iron deficiency
- **B.** false teeth
- **C.** poor oral hygiene
- **D.** vitamin deficiency
- **E.** moniliasis

122. Multiple tongue neuromas may be seen with
- **A.** multiple endocrine adenomatosis
- **B.** tuberous sclerosis
- **C.** neurofibromatosis
- **D.** amyloidosis
- **E.** the Sturge–Weber syndrome

123. A 30-year-old woman presents with fever and sore throat. The physical findings predictive of a positive throat culture for group A streptococci include
- **A.** pharyngeal erythema
- **B.** palatal petechiae
- **C.** tonsillar exudate
- **D.** tender anterior cervical adenopathy
- **E.** enlarged tonsils

5 The Eye

DIRECTIONS: Each of the questions or incomplete statements below is followed by five suggested answers or completions. Select the **one** that is best in each case.

124. All of the following are correct steps for ophthalmoscopic examination of the right eye EXCEPT
- **A.** sit or stand at the patient's right side
- **B.** hold the ophthalmoscope in the right hand and examine with the right eye
- **C.** dim the ambient light
- **D.** rest the left hand on the patient's forehead and hold the upper eyelid with the thumb
- **E.** have the patient look into the beam of light

125. A patient with angioid streaks and a "plucked chicken" appearance of the skin would be expected to have
- **A.** arachnodactyly
- **B.** weak or absent peripheral pulses
- **C.** multiple bony abnormalities
- **D.** necrobiosis lipoidica diabeticorum
- **E.** telangiectasia of the skin

126. A patient with a Marcus Gunn pupil demonstrates
- **A.** a negative swinging flashlight test
- **B.** paradoxical pupillary dilatation
- **C.** contraction of the ciliary muscle
- **D.** a defect in the efferent limb of the pupillary light reflex
- **E.** paradoxical pupillary constriction

127. The near reflex that allows the eye to focus on near objects includes all of the following EXCEPT
A. visual axis convergence
B. pupillary dilatation
C. contraction of the ciliary muscle
D. thickening of the lens
E. increased refraction of light rays

128. The essential abnormality of hypertensive retinopathy is
A. arteriovenous nicking
B. arteriolar constriction
C. widening of the arteriolar light reflex
D. copper wiring
E. silver wiring

129. A unilateral subconjuctival hemorrnage unassociated with pain or visual changes is
A. suggestive of acute glaucoma
B. usually indicative of thrombocytopenia
C. usually due to arteriolar sclerosis
D. an ocular emergency requiring consultation
E. usually an innocuous, idiopathic event

130. A teenage boy suffers a sudden decrease in visual acuity due to traumatic injury to the eyeball. Physical examination reveals blood in the anterior chamber. This is a
A. hypopyon
B. conjunctival hemorrhage
C. corneal abrasion
D. hyphema
E. vitreous hemorrhage

131. A yellowish-green or golden-brown pigmented corneal ring
A. suggests the diagnosis of hemochromatosis
B. may not be pathognomonic of Wilson's disease
C. is weakly correlated with neurologic involvement in Wilson's disease
D. is easily visualized with the naked eye
E. is present in the early stages of Wilson's disease

132. The characteristic visual field defect seen with a pituitary tumor is
A. a total homonymous hemianopsia
B. a lower homonymous hemianopsia
C. a bitemporal hemianopsia
D. an upper homonymous hemianopsia
E. monocular blindness

133. A patient's visual acuity is noted to be 20/30. This means
A. the patient sees figures at 20 feet which are normally seen from 30 feet
B. the patient sees figures at 30 feet which are normally seen from 20 feet
C. the figures seen at 20 feet subtend an arc of 30 minutes at the eye
D. the patient's vision is two-thirds normal
E. none of the above

134. Multiple, small, light-colored retinal spots are noted on ophthalmoscopic examination. They are scattered diffusely and are not associated with other retinal findings. The most likely diagnosis is
A. old chorioretinitis
B. hypertensive retinopathy
C. diabetic retinopathy
D. drusen
E. retinal arteriolar sclerosis

135. Ophthalmoscopy reveals a large flat-topped hemorrhage. This configuration is seen with
A. superficial intraretinal hemorrhage
B. preretinal hemorrhage
C. deep intraretinal hemorrhage
D. vitreous hemorrhage
E. choroidal hemorrhage

136. The feature of a choroidal melanoma that is most useful in distinguishing it from a benign nevus is its
- **A.** color
- **B.** shape
- **C.** size
- **D.** location
- **E.** elevation above the plane of the retina

137. Retinal venous pulsations
- **A.** are a normal finding
- **B.** indicate increased intracranial pressure
- **C.** are present with retinal vein occlusion
- **D.** are suggestive of glaucoma
- **E.** are not visible at the disk

138. A patients notes the sudden appearance of numerous "floaters" in one eye. A few weeks later he observes the onset of a progressive, peripheral visual field defect. The most likely diagnosis is
- **A.** retinitis pigmentosa
- **B.** a lens dislocation
- **C.** iritis
- **D.** macular degeneration
- **E.** a retinal detachment

139. Pallor of the disk and complete absence of very small peripheral disk vessels strongly suggest the diagnosis of
- **A.** papilledema
- **B.** ophthalmic artery occlusion
- **C.** retinal arteriolar sclerosis
- **D.** optic atrophy
- **E.** a disk coloboma

140. The most common cause of unilateral exophthalmos is
- **A.** an orbital pseudotumor
- **B.** a lymphoma
- **C.** thyroid exophthalmos
- **D.** a dermoid
- **E.** a sinus carcinoma

141. A corneal arcus is

A. a significant coronary risk factor in men more than 50 years of age
B. a significant coronary risk factor in men less than 50 years of age
C. a significant coronary risk factor in men of all ages
D. strongly correlated with obesity
E. strongly correlated with hypertriglyceridemia

142. Chemosis means

A. conjunctivitis
B. hemorrhage into the anterior chamber of the eye
C. conjunctival edema
D. hemorrhage into the sclera
E. periorbital edema

143. Normally, intraocular pressure should NOT exceed

A. 7 mm Hg
B. 11 mm Hg
C. 14 mm Hg
D. 18 mm Hg
E. 22 mm Hg

144. Retinal cotton-wool spots are due to

A. arteriolar occlusion with infarction of nerve fibers
B. primary degeneration of Bruch's membrane
C. a vasculopathy with leakage of plasma
D. a proliferative retinopathy
E. resolution of retinal hemorrhage

145. Unequal pupils that are round, react to light, and react to a near stimulus

A. usually indicate a significant disorder
B. establish the diagnosis of an Argyll Robertson pupil
C. are a forme fruste of Horner's syndrome
D. establish the diagnosis of an Adie's pupil
E. may be a normal variant

146. In a patient with moderately elevated intraocular pressure and normal visual fields, select the risk factor that is most predictive of the subsequent development of visual loss.
A. Older age
B. A family history of glaucoma
C. A large cup-to-disk ratio
D. Myopia
E. Diabetes mellitus

147. An ectropion is often associated with
A. a pterygium
B. an entropion
C. a pinguecula
D. epiphora
E. ptosis

148. A patient is farsighted (hyperopic). When examining this patient with the ophthalmoscope, all of the following may be noted except
A. a small optic disk
B. a "minus" lens is required to visualize the fundus
C. a pink disk
D. small retinal vessels
E. an absent optic cup

149. A chronic, painless 1-cm mass in the eyelid is probably
A. a chalazion
B. a hordeolum
C. a xanthelasma
D. cellulitis
E. blepharitis

150. A fleshy excrescence extending bilaterally from the nasal conjunctiva onto the cornea is
A. a pinguecula
B. a xanthelasma
C. a pterygium
D. a scleral staphyloma
E. an arcus cornea

151. A patient with blue sclerae should be evaluated for
A. hypoxia
B. methemoglobinemia
C. multiple fractures
D. argyria
E. polycythemia

152. A 25-year-old man presents in the emergency room with a red eye. Fluorescein staining reveals a branching corneal ulcer. The most likely diagnosis is
A. a corneal abrasion
B. a corneal foreign body
C. a corneal thermal burn
D. bacterial keratitis
E. a herpes infection

153. A patient is considered legally blind when the best corrected vision is
A. 20/50 or less in the better eye
B. 20/80 or less in the better eye
C. 20/120 or less in the better eye
D. 20/160 or less in the better eye
E. 20/200 or less in the better eye

154. The essential feature of proliferative diabetic retinopathy is
A. cotton-wool spots
B. microaneurysms
C. neovascularization
D. dot and blot hemorrhages
E. retinal edema

155. A patient complains of "floaters." Ophthalmoscopic examination with a +10 lens reveals small, motile, dark flecks. The most likely diagnosis is
A. an aqueous hemorrhage
B. a corneal opacity
C. a retinal detachment
D. a vitreous hemorrhage
E. degenerative changes of the vitreous

156. A 62-year-old business executive suddenly loses vision in the left eye. Ophthalmoscopic examination reveals pallor of the fundus and a cherry-red appearing macula. The most likely diagnosis is

A. a central retinal vein occlusion
B. multiple sclerosis
C. a carotid aneurysm
D. diabetic retinopathy
E. a central retinal artery occlusion

157. A patient notes swelling and tenderness confined within the lateral margin of the left orbit. The most likely diagnosis is

A. a hordeolum
B. dacryocystitis
C. a chalazion
D. dacryoadenitis
E. orbital cellulitis

158. Iritis is diagnosed best

A. by inspection
B. with fluorescein angiography
C. with the ophthalmoscope
D. with the slit lamp
E. with a gonioscope

159. The area of the ocular fundus that should be examined last is the

A. macula
B. optic nerve head
C. physiologic cup
D. vessels
E. background

160. A patient whose eyes are abnormally far apart has

A. hypertelorism
B. prognathism
C. proptosis
D. hypotelorism
E. micrognathia

161. The physical finding that is common to keratitis, iritis, and acute glaucoma is
- **A.** keratitic precipitates
- **B.** corneal haze
- **C.** a dilated pupil
- **D.** circumcorneal or ciliary injection
- **E.** subconjunctival hemorrhage

162. Band keratopathy suggests the diagnosis of
- **A.** syphilis
- **B.** hyperlipidemia
- **C.** aging
- **D.** hypercalcemia
- **E.** Wilson's disease

163. Bilateral yellowish eyelid plaques are probably
- **A.** Meibomian cysts
- **B.** cholesteatoma
- **C.** sebaceous cysts
- **D.** verrucae
- **E.** xanthelasma

164. Eversion of the upper eyelid is especially helpful in examining for
- **A.** conjunctivitis
- **B.** a foreign body
- **C.** keratitis
- **D.** a hordeolum
- **E.** Horner's syndrome

165. A useful screening test in the patient with "dry eyes" is
- **A.** a conjunctival biopsy
- **B.** tonometry
- **C.** the Schirmer test
- **D.** fluorescein staining of the cornea
- **E.** measurement of lysozyme activity

166. With normal ambient light the normal range of pupillary diameter is
A. 1–5 mm
B. 2–6 mm
C. 3–7 mm
D. 4–8 mm
E. 5–9 mm

167. Ophthalmoscopic examination of a teenager reveals a pale fundus with cream-colored vessels. The most likely explanation is
A. albinism
B. poorly controlled diabetes mellitus
C. a normal variant
D. a hyperlipoproteinemia
E. a central retinal artery occlusion

DIRECTIONS: Each of the questions or incomplete statements below is followed by five suggested answers or completions. Select either true (T) or false (F) for **each** option given.

---

168. A patient with nonparalytic strabismus
A. usually notes diplopia
B. has a persistent defect in relative ocular alignment
C. has a normal corneal light reflex
D. is at risk to develop suppression amblyopia
E. often has headaches and reading problems

169. Reflection of light from the cornea may interfere with careful retinal examination. Maneuvers that are useful in minimizing this problem include
A. directing the beam of light toward the edge of the pupil
B. using red-free light
C. using the small aperture on the ophthalmoscope
D. using a slit aperture
E. using a dust cover/polarizing filter

170. Which of the following systemic disorders are associated with bilateral cataracts?
- **A.** Hyperparathyroidism
- **B.** Galactosemia
- **C.** Klinefelter's syndrome
- **D.** Down's syndrome
- **E.** Atopic dermatitis

171. Expected findings with a central retinal vein occlusion include
- **A.** retinal pallor
- **B.** papilledema
- **C.** retinal hemorrhages
- **D.** cotton-wool spots
- **E.** narrowed retinal veins

172. Hard retinal exudates
- **A.** are due to infarcted nerve fibers
- **B.** represent deposition of intraretinal lipoids
- **C.** have discrete borders
- **D.** may be confused with drusen
- **E.** are larger than cotton-wool spots

173. Early ophthalmoscopic findings of papilledema include
- **A.** blurring of optic nerve margins
- **B.** loss of retinal artery pulsations
- **C.** distention of retinal veins
- **D.** very small cotton-wool spots
- **E.** hyperemia of the optic nerve

174. The optic disk
- **A.** appears small after a lens extraction
- **B.** measures 15 mm in diameter
- **C.** usually has a more distinct nasal than temporal margin
- **D.** appears magnified about three times because of the cornea and lens
- **E.** appears small with myopia

175. Flame-shaped retinal hemorrhages
- **A.** are located in the middle retinal layer
- **B.** are frequently seen with hypertension
- **C.** are located in the nerve fiber layer
- **D.** are diagnostic of diabetes mellitus
- **E.** may coalesce to form a large hemorrhagic area

176. The macula
- **A.** usually has a lighter color than the adjacent retina
- **B.** is recognized by the pinpoint elevation of the fovea
- **C.** receives its nutrients from choroidal vessels
- **D.** is located nasal to the disk
- **E.** is about the same size as the disk

177. A Roth spot
- **A.** is usually found on the pads of the fingers
- **B.** is diagnostic of endocarditis
- **C.** may be seen with leukemia
- **D.** is a small retinal hemorrhage with a central white area
- **E.** is a small retinal exudate with a central hemorragic area

178. The physiologic blind spot
- **A.** corresponds to the macula
- **B.** is due to the absence of rods and cones in the optic disk
- **C.** enlarges with papilledema
- **D.** is usually round
- **E.** is located nasal to the point of fixation

179. Retinal microaneurysms suggest the diagnosis of
- **A.** diabetes millitus
- **B.** retinal branch vein occlusion
- **C.** hypertensive retinopathy
- **D.** hereditary retinal degeneration
- **E.** retinal branch artery occlusion

180. A chronically hypertensive patient undergoes an ophthalmoscopic examination. Reversible hypertensive retinal abnormalities that may be present include

A. papilledema
B. arteriovenous nicking
C. hemorrhages
D. exudates
E. widening of the light reflex

181. The correct pairing of extraocular muscles with cardinal positions of gaze is

A. nasal elevation–superior rectus
B. temporal depression–superior oblique
C. lateral deviation–lateral rectus
D. nasal depression–inferior rectus
E. medial deviation–medial rectus

182. Senile macular degeneration

A. has a characteristic ophthalmoscopic appearance
B. is slowly progressive
C. does not cause total blindness
D. affects peripheral vision
E. may be mistaken for systemic disorders

183. Correct statements concerning the use of the ophthalmoscope include

A. minus lenses neutralize myopia
B. plus lenses have red numbers
C. the small round aperture is useful with small pupils
D. the slit beam of light aids in assessing the third dimension of retinal lesions
E. red-free light is useful in distinguishing retinal melanin from hemoglobin

6 General Appearance and Diseases

DIRECTIONS: Each of the questions or incomplete statements below is followed by five suggested answers or completions. Select the **one** that is best in each case.

184. A male college student is not able to adduct the left eye when looking to the right or to adduct the right eye when looking to the left. The most likely diagnosis is

A. diabetes mellitus
B. a brain tumor
C. periarteritis nodosa
D. a cerebral aneurysm
E. multiple sclerosis

185. A mentally retarded patient has wartlike excrescenses on the cheeks and "leaf-shaped" macular lesions on the back. The most likely diagnosis is

A. Sturge–Weber disease
B. von Hippel–Lindau disease
C. cerebral palsy
D. tuberous sclerosis
E. Alzheimer's disease

186. A 30-year-old homosexual male develops a chronic fever. Select the clinical feature that is most confirmatory of the diagnosis of the acquired immunodeficiency syndrome.

A. Diarrhea
B. Red-purple macules and papules
C. Pharyngitis
D. Weight loss
E. Lymphadenopathy

187. A patient presents with dementia and diarrhea. Physical examination reveals diffuse erythema and areas of brown scales on the arms. Glossitis is also present. The most likely diagnosis is

A. pernicious anemia
B. Whipple's disease
C. pellagra
D. beriberi
E. scurvy

188. A 68-year-old patient with thrombocythemia notes burning discomfort in the toes and fingers, which is exacerbated by standing or exposure to heat. The involved areas are erythematous and warm. The most likely diagnosis is

A. arteriosclerosis obliterans
B. Raynaud's disease
C. diabetes mellitus
D. erythromelalgia
E. a functional disorder

189. An indigent patient presents in an emergency room with confusion, bilateral sixth nerve palsies, horizontal nystagmus, and gait ataxia. The most likely diagnosis is

A. multiple sclerosis
B. a subdural hematoma
C. a brain tumor
D. hydrocephalus
E. the Wernicke–Korsakoff syndrome

190. A 45-year-old woman has a hereditary disorder manifest by nail dystrophy and proteinuria. Select the physical finding which is confirmatory of this syndrome.
A. Subcutaneous nodules
B. Cherry angiomata
C. Absent patellae
D. Nasal polyps
E. Clonus

191. A teenage girl is much shorter than her peers. Additional findings include neck webbing and sexual infantilism. The most likely diagnosis is
A. achondroplasia
B. Hurler's syndrome
C. hypopituitarism
D. Turner's syndrome
E. hypothyroidism

192. A large 40-year-old man develops wrinkling of the facial skin, a prominent jaw, and large hands. The most likely diagnosis is
A. gigantism
B. Marfan's syndrome
C. hypertrophic osteoarthropathy
D. acromegaly
E. eunuchoidism

193. A patient with multiple cysts of the face and scalp and an osteoma of the jaw should be evaluated for
A. familial colonic polyposis
B. Peutz–Jegher's syndrome
C. Gardner's syndrome
D. von Recklinghausen's disease
E. Paget's disease

194. A middle-aged woman has a 15-year history of recurrent right upper quadrant pain that radiates to the back. On respiration, a clicking sound is heard over the right costal margin. She has had a cholecystectomy. The most likely diagnosis is
- **A.** a rib fracture
- **B.** periostitis
- **C.** costochondritis
- **D.** the slipping rib syndrome
- **E.** intercostal myositis

195. A 50-year-old woman notes the onset of midline pubic pain. There are no other symptoms. Abdominal, rectal, and pelvic examinations are unremarkable except for tenderness on palpation of the symphysis pubis. The most likely diagnosis is
- **A.** a urinary tract infection
- **B.** pelvic inflammatory disease
- **C.** functional bowel disease
- **D.** osteitis pubis
- **E.** hypertrophic osteoarthropathy

196. A 62-year-old man with diffuse arteriosclerotic vascular disease develops dysarthria and dysphagia. He also demonstrates spontaneous crying. The most likely diagnosis is
- **A.** bulbar palsy
- **B.** pseudobulbar palsy
- **C.** Parkinson's disease
- **D.** multiple sclerosis
- **E.** myasthenia gravis

197. A 55-year-old woman develops severe right lower chest pain and malaise. Because of increasing discomfort, 4 days later she visits her physician. The most helpful physical finding in establishing a specific diagnosis would be
- **A.** splinting
- **B.** right lower chest wall tenderness
- **C.** hypoventilation
- **D.** fever
- **E.** unilateral vesicles in a dermatomal distribution

198. A 40-year-old patient presents with uremia, hematuria, and right and left upper quadrant masses. The most likely diagnosis is

A. the hepatorenal syndrome
B. polycystic kidney disease
C. amyloidosis
D. sarcoidosis
E. a metastatic hypernephroma

199. A 30-year-old woman notes the sudden onset of a high fever, nausea and vomiting, diarrhea, and myalgias. Thereafter she develops diffuse erythroderma, hypotension, and confusion. The most likely diagnosis is

A. the toxic shock syndrome
B. the Kawasaki syndrome
C. the scalded skin syndrome
D. scarlet fever
E. acute rheumatic fever

200. A 50-year-old woman suddenly develops fever and erythematous swelling over the bridge of the nose that extends laterally beneath both eyes. The inflamed area is painful. The most likely diagnosis is

A. lupus erythematosus
B. angioneurotic edema
C. contact dermatitis
D. erysipelas
E. herpes zoster

201. After sexual exposure a 25-year-old male develops a urethral discharge. Thereafter he notes painful swelling of the ankles and hyperkeratotic papules of the soles. The most likely diagnosis is

A. rheumatoid arthritis
B. gonorrhea
C. Reiter's syndrome
D. psoriasis
E. syphilis

202. A 20-year-old male with a history of febrile episodes, painful paresthesias, and proteinuria is noted to have 3-mm, red, telangiectatic papules around the umbilicus and on the scrotum. The most likely diagnosis is

A. hereditary hemorrhagic telangiectasia
B. Fordyce's angiokeratomas
C. senile cherry angiomas
D. Fabry's disease
E. histiocytosis-X

203. A chronically ill 30-year-old man presents with sallow skin, Kussmaul's respiration, confusion, and twitching. The most likely diagnosis is

A. cirrhosis
B. hypothyroidism
C. chronic renal failure
D. hypopituitarism
E. pernicious anemia

204. A 35-year-old dwarf has a normal trunk, short limbs, a prominent lumbar lordosis, a large head, and a saddle nose. This is

A. pituitary dwarfism
B. achondroplasia
C. primordial dwarfism
D. progeria
E. Hurler's syndrome

205. A 50-year-old woman has experienced frequent bouts of intense, lancinating facial pain that lasts a few seconds. The pain is confined to the right cheek and upper lip. Touching the cheek or lip may precipitate the paroxysm of pain. The most likely diagnosis is

A. sinusitis
B. a dental abscess
C. temporomandibular joint dysfunction
D. trigeminal neuralgia
E. atypical facial pain

206. The physical finding most helpful in distinguishing polycythemia vera from secondary polycythemia is
A. hepatomegaly
B. a plethoric facies
C. hypertension
D. splenomegaly
E. retinal venous engorgement

207. An 18-year-old college student develops a fever and a severe sore throat. Physical examination reveals generalized lymphadenopathy, splenomegaly, and palatal petechiae. The most likely diagnosis is
A. a viral pharyngitis
B. infectious mononucleosis
C. toxoplasmosis
D. streptococcal pharyngitis
E. gonococcal pharyngitis

208. A patient's neck is noted to be broad and short, and there is decreased range of neck motion. Additional physical findings include low-set ears and a low hairline. The most likely diagnosis is
A. Down's syndrome
B. Turner's syndrome
C. Hurler's syndrome
D. Klippel–Feil syndrome
E. Riley–Day syndrome

209. A 72-year-old man develops severe headaches, fever, and decreased visual acuity. A specific physical finding that should be sought is
A. sinus tenderness
B. an inflamed tympanic membrane
C. spasm of the neck muscles
D. indurated, tender temporal arteries
E. increased intraocular pressure

210. A young woman is noted to have anisocoria. The enlarged pupil reacts slowly to light and accommodates slowly. Deep tendon reflexes are also absent. No other abnormalities are noted. The most likely diagnosis is

A. an intracranial aneurysm
B. diabetes mellitus
C. syphilis
D. a brain tumor
E. Adie's syndrome

DIRECTIONS: Each of the questions or incomplete statements below is followed by five suggested answers or completions. Select either true (T) or false (F) for **each** option given.

---

211. Typical features of an adult with prepubertal eunuchoidism include

A. a normal height
B. an arm span greater than height
C. normal pubic hair
D. a high-pitched voice
E. an upper body segment longer than the lower body segment

212. A woman develops hirsutism. Physical findings that suggest the additional diagnosis of virilization include

A. deepening of the voice
B. weight gain
C. alopecia areata
D. clitoral hypertrophy
E. breast atrophy

213. The physical examination is especially valuable for

A. assessing the severity of illness
B. detecting valvular heart disease
C. defining an intracranial mass
D. detecting a testicular mass
E. appreciating respiratory distress

214. The patient's facies may suggest a specific diagnosis in which of the following disorders?

A. Diabetes mellitus
B. Parkinson's disease
C. Cushing's syndrome
D. Graves' disease
E. Hypothyroidism

215. Characteristic clinical features of an adult with Down's syndrome include

A. Brushfield's spots
B. a normal stature
C. a small tongue
D. small fifth fingers
E. a single transverse palmar crease, bilaterally

7 The Genitalia

DIRECTIONS: Each of the questions or incomplete statements below is followed by five suggested answers or completions. Select the **one** that is best in each case.

---

216. A varicocele is a scrotal mass that
A. can be transilluminated
B. usually occurs on the right side
C. is less apparent in the supine position
D. commonly occurs bilaterally
E. may be easily confused with a hydrocele

217. The most striking characteristic of early prostatic carcinoma on physical examination is its
A. rapid enlargement
B. nodularity
C. tenderness
D. fluctuance
E. induration

218. Cervical cysts are noted while performing a Papanicolaou test. The most likely diagnosis is
A. a Bartholin cyst
B. Nabothian follicles
C. cervical erosions
D. a cervical polyp
E. a cervical carcinoma

219. A woman with a profuse, greenish, bubbly vaginal discharge is noted to have red spots on the cervix. The most likely diagnosis is

A. *Trichomonas* vaginitis
B. *Candida* vaginitis
C. senile vaginitis
D. gonococcal vaginitis
E. *Corynebacterium* vaginitis

220. A painless testicular mass suggests the diagnosis of

A. epididymitis
B. testicular torsion
C. an epididymal cyst
D. a spermatocele
E. a testicular carcinoma

221. Bulging of the distal posterior vaginal wall into the introitus is

A. a rectocele
B. a cystocele
C. an enterocele
D. a urethrocele
E. a uterine descensus

222. A 20-year-old man develops an indurated, painless ulcer of the prepuce. The next step in the evaluation of this lesion should be to

A. obtain a biopsy specimen from the lesion
B. perform a serological test for syphilis
C. treat with penicillin and document the response
D. Gram stain the lesion
E. perform a dark-field examination

223. A spermatocele is usually found

A. in the epididymis
B. attached to the vas deferens
C. as an appendage to the tunica vaginalis
D. in the ejaculatory duct
E. in the testicle

224. What percent of prostatic carcinoma is found in the gland's posterior lobe?
A. 10%
B. 25%
C. 40%
D. 60%
E. 75%

225. The most accurate method for diagnosing testicular torsion is
A. palpation
B. palpation after a spermatic cord block
C. use of the Doppler ultrasonic stethoscope
D. use of a nuclear scan
E. use of ultrasonography

226. Examination of an infertile 26-year-old man demonstrates hypospadias, small testicles, and gynecomastia. The most likely diagnosis is
A. Kleinfelter's syndrome
B. Reifenstein's syndrome
C. Kallmann's syndrome
D. hypopituitarism
E. eunuchoidism

227. A 55-year-old man notes a "lump" on the shaft of his penis and the development of penile "bowing" during erection. The most likely diagnosis is
A. a carcinoma
B. a traumatic hematoma
C. a paraphimosis
D. Peyronie's disease
E. a priapism

228. A verrucous, moist growth on the glans penis suggests the diagnosis of
A. condyloma latum
B. condyloma acuminatum
C. chancroid
D. a chancre
E. a carcinoma

229. A patient notes a few yellow, 1-cm scrotal wall nodules. The most likely diagnosis is
- **A.** a hyperlipidemia
- **B.** a carcinoma
- **C.** candidiasis
- **D.** sebaceous cysts
- **E.** lymphoceles

230. A patient with sickle-cell anemia develops a persistent, painful erection. This is
- **A.** a chordee
- **B.** Peyronie's disease
- **C.** a priapism
- **D.** a phimosis
- **E.** a paraphimosis

231. A 28-year-old woman notes irregular vaginal bleeding and pelvic pain. Pelvic examination suggests a "fullness" in the right oviduct. Which diagnosis must be EXCLUDED?
- **A.** An endometrial carcinoma
- **B.** An ectopic pregnancy
- **C.** A cervical carcinoma
- **D.** Endometriosis
- **E.** Acute salpingitis

232. A 22-year-old woman presents in the emergency room with severe pain involving the genitalia. Examination reveals numerous vesicles of the labia and cervix. The most likely diagnosis is
- **A.** herpes simplex
- **B.** gonorrhea
- **C.** pediculosis pubis
- **D.** erysipelas
- **E.** syphilis

233. Movement of the cervix produces exquisite pain in a 30-year-old woman with lower abdominal pain and fever. This suggests the diagnosis of
A. cystitis
B. vaginitis
C. pelvic peritonitis
D. uterine fibroids
E. a cervical carcinoma

234. The condition in which the prepuce cannot be retracted over the glans penis is
A. a chordee
B. a priapism
C. a phimosis
D. a paraphimosis
E. balanitis

235. A 60-year-old woman develops postmenopausal vaginal bleeding. She should
A. be reexamined in 1 month
B. have a hysterectomy
C. receive a Papanicolaou test
D. have a dilatation and curettage
E. receive a vaginal culture

236. The most sensitive screening tool for prostatic cancer is
A. the digital rectal examination
B. a radioimmunoassay for acid phosphatase
C. urine cytology
D. ultrasonography
E. computed tomography

237. A 50-year-old man presents with a scrotal mass. Auscultation over the mass reveals bowel sounds. This establishes the diagnosis of
A. epididymitis
B. a hydrocele
C. a varicocele
D. a scrotal hernia
E. a spermatocele

238. An obese 40-year-old woman develops right groin pain and bulging of the right labium majora. The most likely diagnosis is

- **A.** a femoral hernia
- **B.** an inguinal hernia
- **C.** inguinal adenopathy
- **D.** a femoral artery aneurysm
- **E.** lymphedema

DIRECTIONS: Each of the questions or incomplete statements below is followed by five suggested answers or completions. Select either true (T) or false (F) for **each** option given.

---

239. Which of the following is a correct description of structures evaluated during the pelvic examination?

- **A.** The normal clitoris measures approximately 1.5 cm in length
- **B.** The oviduct is normally large enough to be palpated
- **C.** The external cervical os measures approximately 3–5 mm
- **D.** The normal uterus is approximately 15 cm in length
- **E.** The normal ovary is approximately 2.5–3.5 cm in length

240. Which of the following statements about the testicle are correct?

- **A.** The normal mean testicular length is 6.0 cm
- **B.** The right testicle normally hangs lower than the left testicle
- **C.** The normal mean testicular width is 2.5 cm
- **D.** The long testicular axis is in a vertical position
- **E.** Demonstrable fluid is normally present around the testicle

241. A woman's uterus is noted to be enlarged on routine pelvic examination. Uterine physical findings suggestive of the diagnosis of fibroids include
A. symmetrical enlargement
B. nodular enlargement
C. mobility
D. fixation
E. firm texture

242. Bluish discoloration of the cervix may be seen with
A. a cervical erosion
B. pregnancy
C. congestive heart failure
D. a pelvic tumor
E. a localized cervical carcinoma

243. On pelvic examination a 30-year-old woman's cervix is not easily moved from side to side. This may be seen with
A. a carcinoma
B. endometriosis
C. obesity
D. retrodisplacement of the uterus
E. pelvic inflammatory disease

244. Which of the following abnormalities occur more commonly in young women with prenatal exposure to diethylstilbestrol than in controls?
A. Transverse vaginal ridges
B. Enlarged ovaries
C. Vaginal adenosis
D. Cervical erosions
E. Clear-cell adenocarcinoma of the vagina

245. A 45-year-old man notes a scrotal mass. Transillumination is especially helpful in diagnosing a
A. varicocele
B. hernia
C. hydrocele
D. testicular tumor
E. spermatocele

8 The Head and Neck

DIRECTIONS: Each of the questions or incomplete statements below is followed by five suggested answers or completions. Select the **one** that is best in each case.

246. A patient has been hoarse for 4 weeks. The most important step in evaluating this problem is

A. a throat culture
B. inspection of the pharynx
C. palpation and transillumination of the sinuses
D. inspection of the tympanic membranes
E. laryngoscopy

247. According to a cephalad–caudad orientation, which of the following is the correct listing of midline neck structures?

A. Hyoid cartilage, cricoid cartilage, thyroid cartilage, isthmus of the thyroid
B. Thyroid cartilage, hyoid cartilage, cricoid cartilage, isthmus of the thyroid
C. Cricoid cartilage, isthmus of the thyroid, hyoid cartilage, thyroid cartilage
D. Hyoid cartilage, thyroid cartilage, cricoid cartilage, isthmus of the thyroid
E. Thyroid cartilage, cricoid cartilage, hyoid cartilage, isthmus of the thyroid

248. The feature most helpful in distinguishing the thyroid gland from other neck masses is its
A. location
B. consistency
C. size
D. upward movement on swallowing
E. shape

249. A tracheal tug suggests the diagnosis of
A. an aortic aneurysm
B. aortic insufficiency
C. a substernal goiter
D. an enlarged pyramidal lobe of the thyroid
E. mediastinal fibrosis

250. All of the following causes of a unilateral cervical mass can be suspected from the physical examination of the neck EXCEPT
A. a lymphoma
B. a branchial cleft cyst
C. a cystic hygroma
D. a carotid body tumor
E. a laryngocele

251. The most distinctive diagnostic feature of a thyroglossal duct cyst is
A. definite fluctuation on palpation
B. translucency
C. an upward movement with the thyroid on swallowing
D. an upward tug when the tongue is protruded
E. location in the midline of the neck

252. A thyroid bruit usually suggests the diagnosis of
A. carotid atherosclerosis
B. a thyroid cyst
C. a colloid goiter
D. Graves' disease
E. thyroid cancer

253. A 60-year-old man has an enlarged skull with frontal bossing. The temporal arteries are dilated and bruits are audible over the bone. This suggests the diagnosis of

A. temporal arteritis
B. occult hydrocephalus
C. an arteriovenous malformation
D. Paget's disease
E. acromegaly

254. Which head and neck structure is NOT normally palpable?

A. Submandibular gland
B. Lymph gland
C. Thyroid gland
D. Parotid gland
E. The hyoid bone

DIRECTIONS: Each of the questions or incomplete statements below is followed by five suggested answers or completions. Select either true (T) or false (F) for **each** option given.

---

255. Which of the following statements about the thyroid gland is correct?

A. The normal gland weighs about 40 g
B. The normal adult gland is fixed to the trachea and larynx
C. The normal dimensions of the lateral lobe of the thyroid are about 7 cm × 5 cm × 2 cm
D. The left lobe is normally larger than the right
E. The pyramidal lobe descends toward the mediastinum

256. Clinical features of a thyroid nodule that suggest a malignant etiology include

A. occurrence together with other thyroid nodules
B. fixation of the gland to adjacent structures
C. adjacent lymphadenopathy
D. a hard consistency
E. history of childhood irradiation to the head and neck

257. The differential diagnosis of facial edema includes
A. hypoproteinemia
B. hypothyroidism
C. tricuspid stenosis
D. an allergic reaction
E. trichinosis

9 The Heart and Vessels

DIRECTIONS: Each of the questions or incomplete statements below is followed by five suggested answers or completions. Select the **one** that is best in each case.

---

258. The first heart sound is produced by
- **A.** opening of the atrioventricular valves
- **B.** closure of the aortic and pulmonic valves
- **C.** opening of the aortic and pulmonic valves
- **D.** vibratory events surrounding the closure of the atrioventricular valves
- **E.** vibratory events accompanying the closure of the aortic and pulmonic valves

259. A pulsus alternans suggests the diagnosis of
- **A.** cardiac tamponade
- **B.** heart block
- **C.** bigeminy
- **D.** left ventricular failure
- **E.** hypokalemia

260. Deep vein thrombosis of the calf is
- **A.** identified by a palpable cord
- **B.** identified by local pain and tenderness
- **C.** identified by a positive Homan's test
- **D.** identified by the sphygmomanometer cuff pain test
- **E.** often silent

261. A loud S_1 is heard with
- **A.** emphysema
- **B.** cardiac failure
- **C.** a short PR interval
- **D.** obesity
- **E.** a pericardial effusion

262. The jugular veins may be used as a manometer to estimate right atrial pressure. Select the INCORRECT statement about this process.
- **A.** The pressure is usually expressed as centimeters of vertical venous distention or undulation above a reference point
- **B.** The reference point for expressing jugular venous pressure is usually the sternal angle of Louis
- **C.** Jugular venous distention (or undulation) is normally less than 9 cm above the right atrium
- **D.** The measurement of jugular venous pressure is usually made is the supine position
- **E.** The measurement of jugular venous pressure can be made employing either the distended external jugular vein or the undulating internal jugular vein

263. Cyclic variation of the heart rate with respiration is
- **A.** a pulsus paradoxus
- **B.** a sinus arrhythmia
- **C.** a pulsus alternans
- **D.** suggestive of cardiac tamponade
- **E.** Kussmaul's sign

264. A useful characteristic in distinguishing the murmur of tricuspid stenosis from that of mitral stenosis is
- **A.** inspiratory augmentation
- **B.** presystolic accentuation
- **C.** a diastolic thrill
- **D.** a sternal lift
- **E.** a low-pitched quality

265. All of the following are high-pitched sounds EXCEPT
A. an S_4
B. a split S_1
C. a systolic ejection sound
D. an opening snap
E. a systolic click

266. An S_4 is frequently found in patients with all the following conditions EXCEPT
A. hypertension
B. atrial fibrillation
C. aortic stenosis
D. a cardiomyopathy
E. coronary artery disease

267. Physical examination of a patient experiencing angina pectoris may reveal all of the following EXCEPT
A. normal physical findings
B. an S_3 gallop
C. an S_4 gallop
D. paradoxical splitting of S_2
E. a transient diastolic rumble

268. A patient with severe chest pain is noted to clench his fist over the sternum while describing the pain. This suggests the diagnosis of
A. atherosclerotic coronary artery disease
B. esophageal spasm
C. a pulmonary infarction
D. pneumonia
E. pericarditis

269. The "a" wave of the jugular venous pulse is produced by
A. atrial diastole
B. rapid ventricular filling
C. opening of the atrioventricular valves
D. transmission of the carotid impulse
E. atrial contraction

270. Select the incorrect statement about the normally functioning prosthetic mitral (ball) valve.
- **A.** The mitral valve opening sound is louder than the closure sound
- **B.** A low-pitched diastolic murmur is often present
- **C.** The accompanying systolic ejection murmur is not due to mitral insufficiency
- **D.** The mitral valve closure sound often obscures S_1
- **E.** The timing of the mitral valve opening sound is similar to the opening snap heard with moderate mitral stenosis

271. The postphlebitic syndrome is characterized by all of the following EXCEPT
- **A.** increased pigmentation of the legs
- **B.** cutaneous atrophy
- **C.** dependent rubor
- **D.** dependent edema
- **E.** chronic ulceration

272. A 64-year-old man has suffered an inferior myocardial infarction. Hemodynamically significant right ventricular infarction is excluded by the absence of elevated jugular venous pressure and
- **A.** pulmonary rales
- **B.** Kussmaul's sign
- **C.** a holosystolic murmur
- **D.** a left-sided S_3
- **E.** a left-sided S_4

273. A continuous, right-sided cervical murmur that disappears with light compression of the internal jugular vein is due to
- **A.** an arteriovenous fistula
- **B.** a patent ductus arteriosus
- **C.** carotid artery stenosis
- **D.** a venous hum
- **E.** an aorticopulmonary window

274. The most likely explanation for the absence of a dorsalis pedis pulse in a 45-year-old asymptomatic male without other physical findings is

A. arteriosclerosis obliterans
B. a coarctation of the aorta
C. Raynaud's disease
D. congenital absence
E. Buerger's disease

275. A 60-year-old man experiences bilateral calf pain after walking one block. Physical examination of the feet reveals a diffuse, persistent red discoloration. The most likely cause of the rubor is

A. ischemic injury
B. erythromelalgia
C. venous insufficiency
D. arteritis
E. atheroembolism

276. A 72-year-old woman experiences syncope. She has a regular heart rate of 36 beats/min. The most likely diagnosis is

A. sinus bradycardia
B. vasovagal syncope
C. a hyperactive carotid sinus
D. a third-degree atrioventricular block
E. hyperventilation

277. A patient demonstrates distended, nonpulsatile neck veins in the erect position. This suggests the diagnosis of

A. tricuspid stenosis
B. tricuspid regurgitation
C. cor pulmonale
D. a third degree atrioventricular block
E. the superior vena caval syndrome

278. A patient with chest pain is noted to have coarse, precordial, scratchy sounds in both systole and diastole. The most likely diagnosis is

A. pneumonia
B. pericarditis
C. a pulmonary infarction
D. an aortic aneurysm
E. mediastinal emphysema

279. Based on phonocardiographic data, select the incorrect statement about ejection murmurs.

A. They are produced by forward flow of blood
B. They are midsystolic in timing
C. Their intensity is crescendo–decrescendo
D. Aortic ejection murmurs terminate prior to A_2
E. Pulmonic ejection murmurs terminate prior to P_2

280. The physical finding that is most suggestive of right ventricular enlargement is

A. an S_3 gallop
B. a right pleural effusion
C. a left parasternal lift
D. a pulsus alternans
E. a diffuse apical impulse

281. An asymptomatic 60-year-old man demonstrates a systolic pulmonary ejection murmur, a loud and delayed tricuspid valve closure sound, and a decreased anterior–posterior transthoracic diameter. The most likely diagnosis is

A. the straight-back syndrome
B. pectus excavatum
C. an atrial septal defect
D. pulmonic stenosis
E. cor pulmonale

282. The murmur of mitral valve prolapse characteristically occurs in

A. early systole
B. midsystole
C. late systole
D. early diastole
E. late diastole

283. Which of the following is the correct relationship of the angle of Louis to the right atrium?
- **A.** It is at the level of the midright atrium
- **B.** It is 5 cm below the level of the midright atrium
- **C.** It is 5 cm above the level of the midright atrium
- **D.** It is 10 cm above the level of the midright atrium
- **E.** It is 15 cm above the level of the midright atrium

284. The following statements concerning the external jugular vein are correct EXCEPT
- **A.** the external jugular vein may not be apparent with increased venous tone
- **B.** the external jugular vein is often occluded in cardiac patients
- **C.** the external jugular vein valves may interfere with retrograde transmission of pressure
- **D.** the external jugular vein is obscured by the sternocleidomastoid muscle
- **E.** local kinking is more likely in the external jugular vein than in the internal system

285. The bell of the stethoscope is particularly useful for auscultating
- **A.** systolic murmurs
- **B.** diastolic murmurs
- **C.** high-pitched sounds
- **D.** low-pitched sounds
- **E.** systolic clicks

286. The internal jugular venous pulse may be distinguished from the carotid arterial pulse by all of the following EXCEPT its
- **A.** multiphasic quality
- **B.** distention with gentle compression
- **C.** change with respiration
- **D.** change with body position
- **E.** location

287. Extremely severe, central chest pain that radiates to the back and is not aggravated by changes in position or respiration suggests the diagnosis of

A. pleuritis
B. a pulmonary infarction
C. an aortic aneurysm with dissection
D. pericarditis
E. an esophageal rupture

288. All of the following support the diagnosis of atrial fibrillation EXCEPT

A. an irregularly irregular rhythm
B. variable intensity of S_1
C. a pulse deficit
D. variable amplitude of the peripheral pulses
E. giant jugular vein "a" waves

289. A 30-year-old, cigarette-smoking male develops migratory thrombophlebitis and claudication of the instep. The most likely diagnosis is

A. a pancreatic carcinoma
B. erythromelalgia
C. Raynaud's disease
D. arteriosclerosis obliterans
E. thromboangitis obliterans

290. An ambulatory patient with organic heart disease has recently gained weight. Which site should be examined first to detect minimal pitting edema?

A. Posterior to the lateral malleolus
B. The anterior tibia
C. The posterior sacral area
D. Posterior to the medial malleolus
E. The dorsum of the foot

291. The chief value of cardiac percussion is to

A. determine visceral situs
B. locate the left heart border
C. estimate cardiac chamber size
D. confirm the presence of a pericardial effusion
E. locate the right heart border

292. An asymptomatic patient receives a periodic health examination. He is noted to have asymmetrical radial pulses. The most likely explanation is
A. the subclavian steal syndrome
B. a dissecting aneurysm
C. the thoracic outlet syndrome
D. arterial thrombosis
E. an aberrant radial artery

293. Select the correct statement concerning the accuracy of precordial palpation in detecting left ventricular enlargement.
A. An apical impulse greater than 10 cm from the midsternal line indicates left ventricular enlargement
B. An apical impulse lateral to the midclavicular line indicates left ventricular enlargement
C. In the left lateral position, the more lateral the apical impulse, the greater the left ventricular size
D. In the left lateral decubitus position, an apical impulse of less than 3 cm reliably excludes left ventricular enlargement
E. In the left lateral position, an apical impulse greater than 3 cm may indicate left ventricular enlargement

294. The hepatojugular reflux
A. is enhanced by the Valsalva maneuver
B. is elicited by pressing on the liver for 5–10 seconds
C. may be helpful in determining whether the venous pressure is elevated
D. is positive with portal hypertension
E. is carried out with the patient in the supine position

295. A 72-year-old patient with coronary heart disease develops hypertension, azotemia, digital cyanosis, and livedo reticularis. The most likely diagnosis is
A. arteriosclerosis obliterans
B. venous insufficiency of the lower extremities
C. atheroembolism
D. Raynaud's phenomenon
E. nephrosclerosis

296. Within a 1-hour period a 50-year-old postoperative patient develops a painful, cyanotic, edematous right leg. The patient becomes hypotensive and arterial pulses are not palpable. The most likely diagnosis is

A. cellulitis and lymphangitis
B. phlegmasia alba dolens
C. complete iliofemoral thrombosis
D. arterial thrombosis
E. arterial emboli

297. A clinician attempts to decide whether a systolic murmur is due to aortic stenosis or mitral insufficiency. All of the following are more suggestive of mitral regurgitation than aortic stenosis EXCEPT

A. the murmur is louder after a premature ventricular depolarization
B. the carotid upstroke is brisk
C. S_1 is masked by the murmur
D. S_2 is normal
E. an apical thrill is audible

298. A patient with a left parasternal lift and a loud S_1 should be suspected of having

A. mitral stenosis
B. tricuspid stenosis
C. pulmonic stenosis
D. multiple pulmonary emboli
E. primary pulmonary hypertension

299. The clinical feature of aortic insufficiency most helpful in distinguishing it from pulmonic insufficiency is

A. a diastolic murmur audible along the left sternal border
B. associated left ventricular enlargement
C. an associated murmur of mitral stenosis
D. a loud S_2
E. bounding peripheral pulses

300. The diagnosis of angina pectoris is established by
A. performing coronary arteriography
B. interviewing the patient
C. auscultating the heart
D. obtaining an exercise electrocardiogram
E. obtaining a resting electrocardiogram

301. Which of the following features is most helpful in identifying chest pain due to myocardial ischemia?
A. Its substernal location
B. Its severe intensity
C. Its radiation down the left arm
D. Its precipitation by exertion
E. Its relief after taking nitroglycerin

302. A patient's holosystolic and rumbling diastolic murmurs vary with positional changes. This suggests the diagnosis of
A. infective endocarditis
B. mitral stenosis and insufficiency
C. tricuspid stenosis and insufficiency
D. an atrial myxoma
E. marantic endocarditis

303. Paradoxical splitting of S_2 is characterized by audible splitting
A. during inspiration with A_2 preceding P_2
B. during expiration with P_2 preceding A_2
C. during inspiration with P_2 preceding A_2
D. during expiration with A_2 preceding p_2
E. heard only with the bell of the stethoscope

304. A grade 3 murmur is
A. prominent but not loud
B. faint but readily heard
C. heard only after concentrated listening
D. loud
E. very loud

305. The single most important physical examination maneuver for establishing the diagnosis of peripheral arterial occlusive disease is
- **A.** observation
- **B.** percussion
- **C.** auscultation
- **D.** palpation
- **E.** a compression test

306. A 35-year-old woman has noted chronic, progressive swelling of the lower extremities. Examination reveals swelling of the toes, feet, and lower legs that does not pit. The skin appears normal except for early verrucous changes. The most likely diagnosis is
- **A.** primary lymphedema
- **B.** chronic venous insufficiency
- **C.** myxedema
- **D.** lipodystrophy
- **E.** chronic panniculitis

307. The thrill of aortic stenosis is best appreciated
- **A.** at the second left interspace in the supine position
- **B.** along the right sternal border in the supine position
- **C.** at the apex in the erect position
- **D.** along the left sternal border in the supine position
- **E.** at the second interspace (left and right) with the patient leaning forward in expiration

308. A pulsus paradoxus is usually demonstrated by
- **A.** placement of an arterial line
- **B.** palpation of the radial pulse
- **C.** use of a sphygmomanometer and stethoscope
- **D.** observation of the neck veins
- **E.** none of the above

309. Which of the following is NOT seen with acute, peripheral arterial occlusion?
A. Pain
B. Edema
C. Coolness
D. Loss of motor function
E. Pallor

310. Innocent systolic murmurs are usually considered to arise in the pulmonic valve, but they may also arise in the
A. bronchial arteries
B. aortic valve
C. pericardium
D. mitral valve
E. tricuspid valve

311. In American adults over the age of 45 years, the prevalence of carotid artery bruits is estimated to be approximately
A. 0.5%
B. 1%
C. 2%
D. 4%
E. 10%

312. A teenage boy is found to have a supraclavicular systolic murmur that almost disappears when the shoulders are hyperextended. This is due to
A. coarctation of the aorta
B. pulmonary stenosis
C. aortic stenosis
D. carotid artery stenosis
E. a functional phenomenon

313. Which is the correct statement concerning the sphygmomanometer bladder size?
- **A.** A 12–14 cm bladder width is appropriate for all adults
- **B.** A bladder width equal to 40% of the midarm diameter is recommended for adults
- **C.** The bladder should be 20 cm in length
- **D.** The length of the bladder should be three times its width
- **E.** The width of the bladder should equal 40% of the midarm circumference

314. Pericardial rubs are heard best
- **A.** along the right sternal border
- **B.** at the lower left sternal border
- **C.** at the apex
- **D.** over the manubrium
- **E.** midway between the apex and base of the heart

315. A 40-year-old woman has a long history of nonexertional chest pain, palpitations, lightheadedness, and fatigue. Physical examination reveals only a midsystolic click. The most likely diagnosis is
- **A.** an anxiety reaction
- **B.** chronic pericarditis
- **C.** papillary muscle dysfunction
- **D.** mitral valve prolapse
- **E.** aortic stenosis

316. The most common cause of a single S_2 is
- **A.** an inaudible A_2
- **B.** an inaudible P_2
- **C.** aortic stenosis
- **D.** Eisenmenger's complex
- **E.** transposition of the great arteries

317. Early diastolic sounds include all of the following EXCEPT
- **A.** an opening snap
- **B.** a pericardial knock
- **C.** a "tumor plop"
- **D.** an S_3
- **E.** a mitral prosthetic sound

318. All of the following are generally considered pathological murmurs EXCEPT
A. late systolic
B. midsystolic
C. holosystolic
D. early diastolic
E. holodiastolic

319. The murmur of a patent ductus arteriosus is characteristically
A. holodiastolic
B. constant in intensity
C. continuous
D. loudest during midsystole
E. easily audible throughout systole and diastole

320. The auscultatory features of acute severe aortic insufficiency differ from those of chronic severe aortic insufficiency in all of the following ways EXCEPT
A. intensity
B. pitch
C. duration
D. tone
E. onset with A_2

321. All of the following may be associated with a lateral displacement of the apical impulse in the absence of organic heart disease EXCEPT
A. pectus excavatum
B. pregnancy
C. an elevated left hemidiaphragm
D. congenital absence of the pericardium
E. pectus carinatum

DIRECTIONS: Each of the questions or incomplete statements below is followed by five suggested answers or completions. Select either true (T) or false (F) for **each** option given.

322. When performing cardiac auscultation, the patient should be routinely examined
A. in the supine position
B. in the sitting or standing position
C. after exercise
D. in the left lateral decubitus position
E. in the right lateral decubitus position

323. Palpation of the carotid artery reveals a double arterial impulse. The first wave is noted in systole, and the second wave is noted in diastole. The differential diagnosis for this observation includes
A. idiopathic cardiomyopathy
B. the febrile state
C. a normal variant
D. cardiac tamponade
E. combined aortic stenosis and insufficiency

324. The third heart sound
A. is also known as an atrial gallop
B. is frequent in normal children
C. may be produced by both the left and right ventricle
D. usually indicates organic heart disease in older adults
E. occurs prior to the opening snap

325. Manifestations of aortic insufficiency include
A. diastolic head nodding
B. visible capillary pulsations
C. Duroziez's murmur
D. a tracheal tug
E. an Austin Flint diastolic murmur

326. In adult coarctation of the aorta
- **A.** the zone of narrowing is usually distal to the origin of the left subclavian artery
- **B.** the blood pressure in the leg is greater than in the arm
- **C.** the femoral pulse is delayed and weak
- **D.** the upper torso may appear athletic while the legs appear thin
- **E.** there is a decreased pulse pressure

327. Palpable, beat-to-beat variations in peripheral pulse strength may be seen with
- **A.** a bifid pulse
- **B.** a pulsus bigeminus
- **C.** atrial fibrillation
- **D.** a sinus arrhythmia
- **E.** a pulsus alternans

328. The pulsus paradoxus may be seen with
- **A.** asthma
- **B.** constrictive pericarditis
- **C.** pulmonary emphysema
- **D.** cardiac tamponade
- **E.** shock

329. Which of the following are features that characterize an innocent cardiac murmur?
- **A.** It is diastolic
- **B.** It is pansystolic
- **C.** It is grade 3 or less
- **D.** It is associated with abnormal splitting of the second heart sound
- **E.** It is heard best at the pulmonic area

330. The major Jones criteria for making the diagnosis of rheumatic fever include
- **A.** erythema nodosum
- **B.** carditis
- **C.** chorea
- **D.** subcutaneous nodules
- **E.** arthralgias

331. A young woman notes painful changes in the color of her fingers with cold exposure. After a careful evaluation and follow-up no underlying medical problem is identified.
- **A.** The sequential color changes are pallor, cyanosis, and erythema, respectively
- **B.** The sequential color changes are erythema, pallor, and cyanosis, respectively
- **C.** She has Raynaud's disease
- **D.** She has Raynaud's phenomenon
- **E.** She will likely develop finger ulcerations

332. A precordial thrill
- **A.** is best timed by auscultation
- **B.** may be a normal variant
- **C.** is a palpable organic murmur
- **D.** is often palpable before a murmur is audible
- **E.** accompanies most murmurs

333. Essential positions for auscultating a faint mitral stenosis murmur include the
- **A.** apex as the patient moves into the left lateral position
- **B.** apex after exercise
- **C.** fourth left interspace in the supine position
- **D.** second left interspace in the erect position
- **E.** apex in the left lateral position

334. While a patient is performing a sustained Valsalva maneuver the
- **A.** cardiac output falls
- **B.** systemic arterial blood pressure increases
- **C.** heart rate increases
- **D.** pulse pressure widens
- **E.** murmurs of idiopathic hypertrophic subaortic stenosis and mitral valve prolapse may increase in intensity

335. An S_1 of varying intensity would be expected with
- **A.** a complete heart block
- **B.** a first degree heart block
- **C.** a right bundle branch block
- **D.** atrial fibrillation
- **E.** ventricular tachycardia

336. The opening snap
A. follows S_3 in diastole
B. is produced by closure of the atrioventricular valves
C. is of shorter duration and is higher pitched than a gallop
D. may be heard with an atrial tumor
E. may be heard with tricuspid stenosis

337. A systolic ejection click
A. may result from the abrupt opening of the semilunar valves
B. may result from sudden distention of the aorta or pulmonary artery
C. may be a normal sound
D. indicates organic heart disease
E. may be affected by respiration

338. Physical findings that may point to a specific cause of chest pain include
A. a pericardial rub
B. a systolic click and late systolic murmur
C. decreased range of motion of the cervical spine
D. left parasternal chest tenderness
E. hyperventilation

339. Physiological splitting of S_2
A. is due in part to an earlier A_2
B. is due in part to a delayed P_2
C. is normally heard at the apex
D. is normal in expiration in the sitting position
E. occurs because of asynchronous closure of the atrioventricular valves

340. The murmur of aortic stenosis
A. increases in intensity as the degree of stenosis increases
B. may be heard better at the apex than at the base of the heart
C. often radiates into the neck
D. is usually heard best in the second left interspace
E. terminates with A_2

341. Pulsus parvus is seen
- **A.** in the normal state
- **B.** with aortic stenosis
- **C.** with mitral stenosis
- **D.** with acute left ventricular failure
- **E.** with cardiac tamponade

342. A palpable apical impulse is usually felt in
- **A.** patients with aortic stenosis
- **B.** normal older adult patients
- **C.** patients with severe hypertension
- **D.** patients with pericardial tamponade
- **E.** normal younger adult patients

343. Kussmaul's sign
- **A.** may be positive with diabetic ketoacidosis
- **B.** is an expiratory increase in jugular venous distention
- **C.** is diagnostic of constrictive pericarditis
- **D.** may be positive with severe right ventricular failure
- **E.** may be positive with a restrictive cardiomyopathy

344. Characteristic physical findings in a patient with chronic constrictive pericarditis include
- **A.** ascites
- **B.** pulmonary edema
- **C.** prominent cardiomegaly
- **D.** a poorly defined apical impulse
- **E.** hepatomegaly

345. Allen's compression test is useful for demonstrating occlusive disease of the
- **A.** subclavian artery
- **B.** brachial artery
- **C.** radial artery
- **D.** ulnar artery
- **E.** palmar arterial arch

346. Preferred methods for identifying S_1 include

A. identifying the sound that is synchronous with the apical impulse

B. listening at the base of the heart where S_1 is softer than S_2

C. identifying the sound that occurs just prior to the upstroke of the carotid artery

D. identifying S_1 by its low pitch

E. identifying the sound that corresponds most closely to the timing of the radial pulse

10 The Lymphatics

DIRECTIONS: Each of the questions or incomplete statements below is followed by five suggested answers or completions. Select the **one** that is best in each case.

347. A 20-year-old man is noted to have an enlarged cervical lymph node. Which clinical finding is of greatest value in deciding whether a biopsy will provide data that will lead to treatment?
A. A lymph node greater than 2 cm in diameter
B. Duration of lymphadenopathy
C. Lymph node tenderness
D. Fever
E. A palpable spleen

348. Focal sternal tenderness has been reported with
A. chronic lymphocytic and myelocytic leukemia
B. acute lymphocytic and myelocytic leukemia
C. severe hemolytic anemia
D. all of the above
E. none of the above

349. The most common presenting manifestation of Hodgkin's disease is
A. fever
B. generalized lymphadenopathy
C. cervical and/or supraclavicular lymphadenopathy
D. hilar lymphadenopathy
E. axillary lymphadenopathy

350. The most common presenting sign with chronic myelocytic leukemia is
A. lymphadenopathy
B. splenomegaly
C. hepatomegaly
D. sternal tenderness
E. purpura

351. Concerning the lymphatic system, all of the following are correct EXCEPT
A. most lymph nodes are palpable
B. shotty inguinal lymph nodes are usually due to inflammation
C. normal young adults may demonstrate palpable posterior cervical nodes
D. periodic lymph node reexamination may be a useful clinical tool
E. epitrochlear lymphadenopathy is usually due to infection

352. Lymph nodes are usually considered to fall within the range of normal size when they measure less than
A. 1.0 cm
B. 1.5 cm
C. 2.0 cm
D. 2.5 cm
E. 3.0 cm

353. Small lymph nodes may be normally palpable in all of the following areas EXCEPT
A. anterior cervical
B. submandibular
C. axillary
D. epitrochlear
E. inguinal

DIRECTIONS: Each of the questions or incomplete statements below is followed by five suggested answers or completions. Select either true (T) or false (F) for **each** option given.

354. Inguinal lymphadenopathy
- **A.** is usually related to localized minor trauma or infection
- **B.** may be secondary to venereal disease
- **C.** is usually clinically significant
- **D.** is usually of less clinical significance than supraclavicular adenopathy
- **E.** is a favored site for node biopsy

355. Carcinomatous lymph nodes are
- **A.** usually very hard
- **B.** often associated with sinus tract formation
- **C.** usually tender on palpation
- **D.** associated with inflamed adjacent skin
- **E.** often bound together and to surrounding tissues

11 The Musculoskeletal System

DIRECTIONS: Each of the questions or incomplete statements below is followed by five suggested answers or completions. Select the **one** that is best in each case.

356. Myoedema is frequently found with
- **A.** diabetes mellitus
- **B.** obesity
- **C.** hypothyroidism
- **D.** hyperparathyroidism
- **E.** Conn's syndrome

357. A middle-aged woman develops painful swelling of her ears and nose, migratory polyarthritis, and iritis. The most likely diagnosis is
- **A.** Wegener's granulomatosis
- **B.** rheumatoid arthritis
- **C.** polyarteritis nodosa
- **D.** relapsing polychondritis
- **E.** scleroderma

358. A 40-year-old woman experiences episodes of sharp pain involving the fourth left toe. Palpation of the third web space demonstrates striking tenderness. The most likely diagnosis is

A. metatarsal osteochondritis
B. a march fracture
C. a plantar neuroma
D. the tarsal tunnel syndrome
E. foot strain

359. A patient with a "tennis elbow" should demonstrate tenderness of the

A. olecranon bursa
B. medial humeral epicondyle
C. lateral humeral epicondyle
D. biceps tendon
E. ulnar nerve at the elbow

360. A short, stocky young woman is noted to have very short fourth metacarpal and metatarsal bones. She should be studied for abnormal metabolism of

A. potassium
B. cholesterol
C. triglyceride
D. magnesium
E. calcium

361. Finkelstein's test is positive with

A. DeQuervain's disease
B. the carpal tunnel syndrome
C. the thoracic outlet syndrome
D. a ganglion
E. degenerative disk disease

362. A cystic, nontender structure located on the dorsum of the hand near the tendon sheaths is probably a

A. ganglion
B. lipoma
C. fibroma
D. rheumatoid nodule
E. tophus

363. Shoulder pain that is exacerbated by flexing and supinating the forearm against resistance suggests the diagnosis of

A. a rotator cuff tear
B. bicipital tendinitis
C. subdeltoid bursitis
D. subcoracoid bursitis
E. pericapsulitis

364. A 22-year-old male notes low back pain and stiffness. He demonstrates reduced flexion of the spine, chest expansion of less than 2.5 cm, and sacroiliac tenderness. The most likely diagnosis is

A. rheumatoid arthritis
B. Scheuermann's disease
C. ankylosing spondylitis
D. low back strain
E. degenerative disk disease

365. In the standing position a woman's knees are noted to be unusually close together while her ankles are abnormally far apart. This is

A. genu valgus
B. genu varus
C. an eversion deformity
D. an equinus deformity
E. cubitus valgus

366. Long, slender fingers are seen in individuals with the following EXCEPT

A. Marfan's syndrome
B. eunuchism
C. Ehlers–Danlos syndrome
D. myxedema
E. an asthenic habitus

367. The joint very rarely involved with osteoarthritis is the

A. distal interphalangeal joint
B. proximal interphalangeal joint
C. metacarpophalangeal joint
D. carpometacarpal joint
E. hip joint

368. A 40-year-old man notes right shoulder pain. Arm abduction is normal up to 60 degrees, but further abduction is painful. There is point tenderness between the greater and lesser humeral tuberosities. The most likely diagnosis is

A. osteoarthritis
B. the "frozen shoulder"
C. chronic supraspinatus tendinitis
D. bicipital tendinitis
E. a complete rupture of the supraspinatus tendon

369. A 50-year-old heavy equipment operator develops severe right buttock pain. Point tenderness is present over the ischial tuberosity. Lateral hip rotation causes pain. The most likely diagnosis is

A. ischiogluteal bursitis
B. spondylolisthesis
C. degenerative disk disease
D. lumbosacral spine strain
E. sacroiliac inflammation

370. Without adequate training, a 38-year-old man runs in a 26-mile race. A few hours thereafter he notes pain over the anterior tibia. The next morning the area is swollen, warm, and erythematous. He is unable to extend the great toe on the involved side. The most likely diagnosis is

A. thrombophlebitis
B. cellulitis
C. lymphangitis
D. the anterior tibial compartment syndrome
E. a tibial stress fracture

371. Measurement of the joint range of motion is accurately achieved by

A. inspecting the joint
B. using a goniometer
C. using a cloth tape measure
D. comparing joints on each side of the body
E. using a ruler

372. Painful fusiform swelling of the proximal interphalangeal joints is most characteristic of
- **A.** rheumatic fever
- **B.** osteoarthritis
- **C.** rheumatoid arthritis
- **D.** gout
- **E.** pseudogout

373. Ballottement of the patella produces a clicking sensation. This is seen with
- **A.** a normal knee
- **B.** synovitis
- **C.** a joint effusion
- **D.** a Baker's cyst
- **E.** bursitis

374. The obturator test is performed with the patient in the supine position by
- **A.** flexing the thigh to 90 degrees, immobilizing the ankle, and moving the knee laterally and medially
- **B.** pressing down on the thigh as the patient elevates the extended leg
- **C.** flexing the knee, placing the foot on the opposite patella, and pushing the knee laterally
- **D.** dorsiflexing the foot with the thigh flexed and the knee extended
- **E.** flexing the thigh maximally and hyperextending the opposite thigh

375. Measurement of leg length should be made from the
- **A.** umbilicus to the lateral malleolus
- **B.** pubic tubercle to the lateral malleolus
- **C.** anterior superior iliac spine to the medial malleolus
- **D.** midinguinal ligament to the medial malleolus
- **E.** anterior superior iliac spine to the lateral malleolus

376. An elderly patient falls and complains of hip pain. Examination of the hip reveals shortening and outward rotation of 90 degrees in the involved limb. This suggests the diagnosis of

A. an intracapsular femoral fracture
B. an extracapsular femoral fracture
C. a lesser trochanteric avulsion fracture
D. a posterior dislocation of the hip
E. an anterior dislocation of the hip

377. Adson's test is performed by palpating

A. the radial pulses with the arms over the head
B. the radial pulses as another examiner forces the shoulders downward and backward
C. for a cervical rib
D. the radial pulses as the patient raises and turns his chin to one side and holds his breath in inspiration
E. the radial pulses as the patient opens and closes his hands

378. A teenage boy notes swelling and tenderness of the right tibial tuberosity. The most likely diagnosis is

A. a tibial fracture
B. an injury of the medial meniscus
C. an infrapatellar fat pad injury
D. an infrapatellar bursitis
E. the Osgood–Schlatter syndrome

379. A middle-aged woman notes knee pain, especially when kneeling. Examination reveals tenderness as the patella is pressed against the condyles and patellar crepitus with joint motion. The most likely diagnosis is

A. the Osgood–Schlatter syndrome
B. chondromalacia of the patella
C. prepatellar bursitis
D. dislocation of the patella
E. rupture of the patellar ligament

380. A teenager injures his right third finger playing baseball. He is unable to extend the distal phalanx of the involved finger. The diagnosis is
A. a mallet finger
B. a trigger finger
C. a typewriter finger
D. a flexor tendon contracture
E. an interphalangeal joint sprain

381. When performing a lumbar puncture, the iliac crests are important landmarks; a line drawn between them passes between the dorsal spines of
A. T-12 and L-1
B. L-1 and L-2
C. L-2 and L-3
D. L-3 and L-4
E. L-4 and L-5

382. A patient's spine is curved to one side and the vertebral bodies are rotated one upon the other. This is a
A. gibbus
B. list
C. kyphosis
D. scoliosis
E. lordosis

383. Recurrent hemarthroses are characteristic of
A. chronic liver disease
B. factor VIII deficiency
C. thrombocytopenia
D. pseudoxanthoma elasticum
E. hereditary hemorrhagic telangiectasia

384. A 50-year-old man develops nodularity of the distal palmar fascia along with flexion contractures of the fourth and fifth fingers. This suggests the diagnosis of
A. a posttraumatic contracture
B. rheumatoid arthritis
C. degenerative arthritis
D. Volkmann's contracture
E. Dupuytren's contracture

DIRECTIONS: Each of the questions or incomplete statements below is followed by five suggested answers or completions. Select either true (T) or false (F) for **each** option given.

---

385. Hypertrophic osteoarthropathy may be characterized by
- **A.** new bone deposition
- **B.** periostitis
- **C.** clubbing
- **D.** synovitis
- **E.** arthritis

386. A popliteal cyst is associated with
- **A.** septic arthritis
- **B.** gout
- **C.** a popliteal artery aneurysm
- **D.** degenerative arthritis
- **E.** rheumatoid arthritis

387. A mentally retarded patient, who is unable to release his grasp after shaking hands, might also be expected to demonstrate
- **A.** cardiomegaly
- **B.** a sensory neuropathy
- **C.** cataracts
- **D.** normal muscle mass and strength
- **E.** testicular atrophy

388. Which of the following statements concerning an unstable knee are correct?
- **A.** An anterior cruciate ligament tear gives a positive posterior drawer sign
- **B.** A posterior cruciate ligament tear gives a positive anterior drawer sign
- **C.** Increased mobility at the knee when abducting the lower leg suggests a lateral collateral ligament injury
- **D.** Increased mobility at the knee when abducting the lower leg suggests a medial collateral ligament injury
- **E.** A lateral collateral ligament injury causes more knee instability than a medial collateral ligament injury

389. Subcutaneous nodules located over bony prominences are seen with
A. Reiter's syndrome
B. rheumatoid arthritis
C. systemic lupus erythematosus
D. degenerative arthritis
E. rheumatic fever

390. Palpation of the temporomandibular joints
A. may be performed anterior to the tragus
B. may reveal crepitation or clicking
C. may be performed through the external auditory canal
D. establishes the diagnosis of dislocation
E. should be done individually

391. Features of "fibrositis" include
A. muscular atrophy
B. trigger points
C. synovitis
D. joint effusions
E. scapular skinfold tenderness

392. Which of the following clinical features are more characteristic of a myopathy than a peripheral neuropathy?
A. Proximal muscle weakness
B. A sensory loss
C. Fasciculations
D. A complete paralysis
E. Early decrease of deep tendon reflexes

393. When using the correct zero starting position, the normal range of motion of the following joints is
A. elbow flexion to 150 degrees
B. knee flexion to 160 degrees
C. ankle dorsiflexion to 40 degrees
D. shoulder abduction to 90 degrees
E. hip extension to 30 degrees

394. Features of carpal spasm include
- **A.** flexion of the thumb on the palm
- **B.** abduction of the fingers
- **C.** wrist flexion
- **D.** metacarpophalangeal joint extension
- **E.** proximal and distal interphalangeal joint extension

395. Objective signs of low back pain include
- **A.** tenderness on palpation
- **B.** loss of lumbar lordosis
- **C.** spasm of the erector spinae
- **D.** a list
- **E.** decreased range of lumbar spine motion

12 The Nervous System

DIRECTIONS: Each of the questions or incomplete statements below is followed by five suggested answers or completions. Select the **one** that is best in each case.

396. The basic or abbreviated neurologic examination should include all of the following EXCEPT examination of
A. pupils, ocular movements, and the ocular fundus
B. tendon and plantar reflexes
C. facial movements and speech
D. the strength of arm and leg muscles
E. cerebellar function

397. In the comatose patient ataxic breathing suggests dysfunction at the level of the
A. medulla
B. cerebral hemispheres
C. diencephalon
D. midbrain
E. pons

398. Amaurosis fugax suggests the diagnosis of
A. hypoglycemia
B. a transient ischemic attack
C. hyperventilation
D. a seizure disorder
E. Meniere's disease

399. A patient with a positive wrist flexion test might be expected to demonstrate all of the following EXCEPT
- **A.** hand pain radiating proximally
- **B.** thenar atrophy
- **C.** a positive Tinel's sign
- **D.** weakened thumb adduction
- **E.** decreased ulnar nerve conduction velocity

400. Decreased or absent deep tendon reflexes are anticipated in conditions affecting all of the following EXCEPT the
- **A.** muscle
- **B.** myoneural junction
- **C.** pyramidal tract
- **D.** peripheral nerve
- **E.** anterior horn cell

401. Numbness and pain develop gradually along the lateral aspect of the thigh. No other abnormalities are noted. The most likely diagnosis is
- **A.** sciatica
- **B.** arteriosclerotic peripheral vascular disease
- **C.** deep vein thrombosis
- **D.** spondylolisthesis
- **E.** meralgia paresthetica

402. With Bell's palsy one expects to see all of the following EXCEPT
- **A.** a smooth brow
- **B.** drooping of the mouth on the involved side
- **C.** a flat nasolabial fold
- **D.** ptosis
- **E.** failure to close the eye

403. A festinating gait suggests the diagnosis of
- **A.** Parkinson's disease
- **B.** Wilson's disease
- **C.** multiple sclerosis
- **D.** tabes dorsalis
- **E.** pernicious anemia

404. Romberg's test primarily evaluates function of the
- **A.** visual system
- **B.** vestibular apparatus
- **C.** cerebellum
- **D.** posterior columns
- **E.** cortical sensory system

405. The neurologic finding that is confirmatory of a pyramidal tract lesion is
- **A.** absent abdominal reflexes
- **B.** decreased deep tendon reflexes
- **C.** decreased muscle tone
- **D.** a flexor plantar reflex
- **E.** fasciculations

406. A noncommunicative elderly patient undergoes neurologic evaluation. The presence of akathisias suggests the patient is receiving
- **A.** chloral hydrate
- **B.** diazepam
- **C.** flurazepam
- **D.** chlorpromazine
- **E.** amitriptyline

407. Asterixis has been associated with all of the following EXCEPT
- **A.** hepatic encephalopathy
- **B.** uremia
- **C.** hypokalemia
- **D.** carbon dioxide retention
- **E.** hyperthyroidism

408. A patient suffers a cardiac arrest and is brought to an emergency room in a comatose state. On initial examination, which clinical feature is most suggestive of virtually no chance of a functional recovery?
- **A.** Absent pupillary light reflexes
- **B.** Nonpurposeful motor responses
- **C.** Failure to open eyes
- **D.** Absence of spontaneous eye movements
- **E.** Absent oculocephalic responses

409. The physical finding most suggestive of carotid artery atherosclerosis is
- **A.** a systolic carotid artery bruit
- **B.** decreased amplitude of the carotid artery pulse
- **C.** a cholesterol embolus in a retinal arteriole
- **D.** hypertension
- **E.** a continuous bruit

410. The first sign of uncal herniation is usually
- **A.** a complete third nerve palsy
- **B.** ipsilateral pupillary dilatation
- **C.** contralateral hemiparesis
- **D.** hemianopsia
- **E.** Cheyne–Stokes respiration

411. Irritation of the first sacral root by a herniated nucleus pulposus might be associated with all of the following EXCEPT
- **A.** posterior thigh pain
- **B.** a positive straight leg raising test
- **C.** hypesthesia of the great toe
- **D.** a decreased Achilles tendon reflex
- **E.** weakness of the plantar flexors

412. A 45-year-old patient presents with the acute onset of low back pain. Physical examination reveals saddle anesthesia, cross-over leg pain, and absent anal sphincter tone. This strongly suggests the diagnosis of
- **A.** acute central disk herniation
- **B.** diabetes mellitus with neuropathy
- **C.** spinal canal stenosis
- **D.** a spinal cord tumor
- **E.** a prostatic carcinoma

413. All of the following tremors are exacerbated by purposeful movement EXCEPT the
- **A.** cerebellar tremor
- **B.** parkinsonian tremor
- **C.** senile tremor
- **D.** hereditary tremor
- **E.** tremor of Wilson's disease

414. Fasciculations are
- **A.** diagnostic of amyotrophic lateral sclerosis
- **B.** not visible with the naked eye
- **C.** only demonstrable with electromyography
- **D.** suggestive of lower motor neuron disease
- **E.** associated with progressive neurological dysfunction

415. With Horner's syndrome all of the following may be seen EXCEPT
- **A.** ptosis
- **B.** mydriasis
- **C.** enophthalmos
- **D.** anhidrosis
- **E.** flushing

416. A nonparalytic disorder characterized by an inability to perform purposeful movements is called
- **A.** agnosia
- **B.** paresis
- **C.** aphasia
- **D.** apraxia
- **E.** hysterical paralysis

417. A patient with a brain tumor is noted to ignore a left-sided hemiplegia and hemianesthesia. The tumor is probably located in the
- **A.** frontal lobe
- **B.** temporal lobe
- **C.** thalamus
- **D.** parietal lobe
- **E.** midbrain

418. A 34-year-old man has a past history of ankle trauma. He presents with painful paresthesias of the forefoot, heel, and calf. Tenderness is demonstrable along the posterior tibial nerve's distribution in the ankle. The most likely diagnosis is
- **A.** an old, unrecognized fracture
- **B.** traumatic arthritis
- **C.** metatarsalgia
- **D.** the tarsal tunnel syndrome
- **E.** reflex sympathetic dystrophy

419. An elderly patient develops weakness. During a neurological examination he is asked to shut his eyes and extend his arms in a supinated position. One arm begins to slowly droop and pronate. This suggests

A. dorsal column disease
B. cerebellar disease
C. a peripheral neuropathy
D. corticospinal tract disease
E. a myopathy

420. Cherry-red skin color in a comatose patient suggests the diagnosis of

A. carbon monoxide poisoning
B. methemoglobinemia
C. polycythemia
D. bacteremia
E. insulin shock

421. A patient is tested for the ability to perform rapid alternating movements. Inability to perform such tests is most likely due to dysfunction of the

A. peripheral nerves
B. cerebellum
C. cerebral cortex
D. myoneural junction
E. muscles

422. Physical examination of a comatose patient reveals an area of ecchymosis over the left mastoid process. Which of the following should be suspected?

A. A subdural hematoma
B. A basilar skull fracture
C. A superficial abrasion
D. An epidural hematoma
E. A coagulopathy

423. A patient who has suffered a cerebrovascular accident is asked to draw a clock. Examination of the drawing reveals that the numbers are crowded on the right side of the clock. This suggests a lesion in the
- **A.** frontal lobe
- **B.** cerebellum
- **C.** temporal lobe
- **D.** parietal lobe
- **E.** occipital lobe

424. The wakeful state is dependent on interaction between the cerebral hemispheres and the
- **A.** cerebellum
- **B.** reticular activating system
- **C.** caudal pons
- **D.** medulla
- **E.** sympathetic nervous system

425. A patient with vertigo undergoes a diagnostic evaluation. His symptoms are reproduced for about 15 seconds after he suddenly assumes the supine position with his head turned to the right or left. Sitting the patient up reverses the direction of the vertigo. This suggests the diagnosis of
- **A.** a cerebellopontine angle tumor
- **B.** multiple sclerosis
- **C.** a brainstem tumor
- **D.** the hyperventilation syndrome
- **E.** benign positional vertigo

426. Nasal speech suggests the diagnosis of
- **A.** paralysis of the soft palate
- **B.** parkinsonism
- **C.** cerebellar dysarthria
- **D.** aphasia
- **E.** pseudobulbar palsy

427. A patient demonstrates a few jerking movements of the eyes on extreme lateral gaze. The most likely diagnosis is
A. nystagmoid movements
B. jerk nystagmus
C. pendular nystagmus
D. rotary nystagmus
E. opticokinetic nystagmus

428. A patient develops rapid, brief, purposeless jerking movements of the right upper extremity. Loud sounds may precipitate the abnormal movements. This is
A. myoclonus
B. chorea
C. dystonia
D. torticollis
E. a tic

429. A patient is taken by his family to a physician because of problems with speech. The patient utters uninterpretable sounds and does not appear to understand written or verbal instructions. This pattern of defective speech is
A. dysarthria
B. aphonia
C. dysphonia
D. aphasia
E. anarthria

430. Kernig's sign is elicited by
A. stroking the lateral plantar surface of the foot
B. passively flexing the head on the chest
C. passively extending one leg on a flexed thigh
D. passively flexing one thigh with the leg in extension
E. passively flexing one leg and thigh

431. A patient with a chronic, broad-based gait cannot perform the heel-to-knee-to-toe test. The most likely diagnosis is
A. cerebellar degeneration
B. pyramidal tract disease
C. hysteria
D. Parkinson's disease
E. a peripheral neuropathy

432. Vertical nystagmus suggests a lesion in the
A. brainstem
B. cerebellum
C. basal nuclei
D. vestibular apparatus
E. eye

433. Evaluation of handedness is especially important in studying
A. aphasia
B. aphonia
C. apraxia
D. anarthria
E. agnosia

434. A patient's tandem gait is almost normal with his eyes open and markedly ataxic with his eyes closed. This is most commonly seen with dysfunction of the
A. cerebellum
B. extrapyramidal tracts
C. peripheral nerves
D. posterior columns
E. vestibular apparatus

435. A lesion that completely destroys the right optic tract produces a
A. right homonymous hemianopsia
B. left homonymous hemianopsia
C. bitemporal hemianopsia
D. binasal hemianopsia
E. right optic atrophy

436. A patient demonstrates involuntary, slow, snakelike movements of the extremities. This is
A. chorea
B. athetosis
C. ballismus
D. dystonia
E. myoclonus

437. The cardinal sign of idiopathic autonomic insufficiency is
A. orthostatic hypotension
B. absence of sinus arrhythmia
C. muscle wasting
D. anhidrosis
E. Horner's syndrome

438. Station is evaluated with the patient
A. sitting on the edge of the examining table
B. standing with the feet several inches apart
C. in the supine position
D. in the prone position
E. standing with the feet close together

439. Chvostek's sign may be positive with all of the following EXCEPT
A. malabsorption
B. hyperventilation
C. hypomagnesemia
D. hypoparathyroidism
E. osteoporosis

440. A comatose patient demonstrates 2–3-second periods of end-inspiratory pauses. Occasional end-expiratory pauses are also noted. This suggests damage in the
A. forebrain
B. pons
C. hypothalamus
D. midbrain
E. medulla

441. Neurological signs that may be seen in normal, aged persons, include all of the following EXCEPT
A. some loss of associated movements
B. vibratory loss in the distal lower extremities
C. spontaneous nystagmus
D. slight terminal finger-to-nose tremor
E. some dorsal interosseous atrophy

442. Vertigo is characterized by a

A. sudden loss of consciousness
B. "lightheaded" sensation
C. sense of "dizziness"
D. rotational sensation
E. sense of dysequilibrium

443. A 65-year-old patient is noted on routine examination to have an asymptomatic carotid bruit. Select the correct statement concerning the natural history of this finding.

A. Prophylactic endarterectomy reduces the likelihood of symptoms or a stroke
B. Patients with a less than 80% diameter reducing lesion may be safely monitored at 6-month intervals with noninvasive methods
C. Stopping smoking has no effect on the likelihood of disease progression
D. Treatment with aspirin and/or dipyridamole reduces the likelihood of disease progression
E. Carotid angiography should be performed on all patients with this finding

444. All of the following are consistent with a lower motor neuron lesion EXCEPT

A. muscular atrophy
B. weakness
C. hyperreflexia
D. fasciculations
E. absent or flexor plantar reflexes

445. Dorsiflexion of the foot produces sustained, rhythmic, alternating flexion and extension. This is

A. a normal variant
B. true clonus
C. pseudoclonus
D. transient clonus
E. suggestive of extrapyramidal tract disease

446. A patient is noted to have a tongue tremor. All of the following may account for this finding EXCEPT

A. anxiety
B. thyrotoxicosis
C. delirium tremens
D. a normal variant
E. Parkinson's disease

447. A 40-year-old man has an abnormal gait that is slow, scuffing, and spastic. His hips adduct very strongly and give a scissorlike quality to the gait. This is a

A. paraplegic gait
B. ataxic gait
C. hemiplegic gait
D. cerebellar gait
E. dystonic gait

448. Testing for meningeal signs is especially important in patients with

A. chronic low back pain
B. fever and neck pain
C. chronic sciatica
D. optic neuritis
E. headaches

449. Lesions of all of the following peripheral nerves are correctly matched with their corresponding deficits EXCEPT

A. long thoracic nerve—winging of the scapula
B. ulnar nerve—claw hand
C. radial nerve—wrist drop
D. tibial nerve—tarsal tunnel syndrome
E. median nerve—interosseous atrophy

DIRECTIONS: Each of the questions or incomplete statements below is followed by five suggested answers or completions. Select either true (T) or false (F) for **each** option given.

450. Tests of cortical sensory function include
- **A.** touch perception
- **B.** two-point discrimination
- **C.** graphesthesia
- **D.** stereognosis
- **E.** vibratory perception

451. Features of decorticate posture include
- **A.** forearm flexion
- **B.** opisthotonos
- **C.** plantar flexion of ankles
- **D.** arm adduction
- **E.** internal rotation of the arms

452. Syringomyelia is characterized by which of the following?
- **A.** Loss of pain and temperature sensation
- **B.** Amyotrophy
- **C.** Trophic ulcers
- **D.** Thoracic scoliosis
- **E.** Preservation of the sense of touch

453. A comatose patient with an intact brainstem would be expected to demonstrate
- **A.** tonic ocular deviation toward the side of cold caloric stimulation
- **B.** absence of doll's eye movement
- **C.** nystagmus toward the side of warm caloric stimulation
- **D.** central neurogenic hyperventilation
- **E.** a ciliospinal pupillary reflex

454. Snout and suck reflexes are
- **A.** always abnormal
- **B.** thought to be due to a release phenomenon
- **C.** seen with coma
- **D.** seen with bilateral frontal lobe disease
- **E.** seen with corticobulbar disease

455. Which of the following deep tendon reflex innervations are correct?
- **A.** Biceps—C5-6
- **B.** Triceps—C6-8
- **C.** Patellar—L5-S1
- **D.** Achilles—S2-4
- **E.** Brachioradialis—C8-T1

456. The corneal reflex
- **A.** is useful for evaluating diplopia
- **B.** may be abnormal with either peripheral or central lesions
- **C.** measures fifth cranial nerve function
- **D.** measures seventh cranial nerve function
- **E.** is intact when only the stimulated eye blinks

457. Persistent deviation of gait to one side suggests
- **A.** hysteria
- **B.** unilateral vestibular disease
- **C.** senility
- **D.** unilateral frontal lobe disease
- **E.** unilateral cerebellar disease

458. The finding of opticokinetic nystagmus
- **A.** is normal when watching a moving object
- **B.** suggests a drug effect
- **C.** suggests a parietal lobe syndrome
- **D.** establishes that a patient is not blind
- **E.** suggests a brainstem lesion

459. Doll's eye movements
- **A.** are absent in the alert adult
- **B.** are present in infants
- **C.** are absent in deep coma
- **D.** indicate brain stem dysfunction in the comatose adult
- **E.** are closely linked to the oculovestibular reflex

460. The Babinski sign
- **A.** consists of a single manifestation—dorsiflexion of the toes
- **B.** consists of a single manifestation—fanning of the toes
- **C.** is an abnormal superficial reflex in adults
- **D.** should be elicited with the knee flexed
- **E.** suggests the presence of extrapyramidal tract disease

461. With neck flexion a patient notes electriclike sensations passing down the body. Which of the following disorders should be suspected?
- **A.** A frontal lobe tumor
- **B.** A protruding cervical disk
- **C.** Hysteria
- **D.** A cervical spine tumor
- **E.** Multiple sclerosis

462. A positive Hoffman sign
- **A.** may be present with tension states
- **B.** is diagnostic of pyramidal tract disease
- **C.** is characterized by abduction of the thumb
- **D.** indicates hypoactive muscle stretch reflexes
- **E.** has the same significance as a positive Babinski sign

463. Which structures are correctly paired with their sensory innervation?
- **A.** The face—cranial nerve V
- **B.** The neck—C-5
- **C.** The nipple—T-5
- **D.** The great toe—S-1
- **E.** The little toe—S-2

464. The "flapping tremor" of hepatic encephalopathy
- **A.** disappears with the development of coma
- **B.** is present at rest
- **C.** is usually bilateral
- **D.** is exacerbated by purposeful movement
- **E.** is exaggerated by sustained posture

465. The consensual light reflex
- **A.** occurs because of semidecussation of optic nerve fibers
- **B.** is absent on the side of a complete third nerve lesion
- **C.** is absent on the side opposite a third nerve lesion
- **D.** is intact in a blind eye if the third nerve is normal
- **E.** is absent on the normal side opposite a blind eye

466. Tests of abstract thinking include
- **A.** reciting multiplication tables
- **B.** the MMPI
- **C.** interpretation of proverbs
- **D.** explanation of similarities between objects
- **E.** interpretation of analogies

13 The Skin

DIRECTIONS: Each of the questions or incomplete statements below is followed by five suggested answers or completions. Select the **one** that is best in each case.

467. Recurrent crops of petechiae are characteristic of
- **A.** thrombocytopenia
- **B.** chronic liver disease
- **C.** von Willebrand's disease
- **D.** hemophilia
- **E.** malnutrition

468. A heliotrope rash involving the upper eyelids is characteristic of
- **A.** trichinosis
- **B.** scleroderma
- **C.** blepharitis
- **D.** seborrheic dermatitis
- **E.** dermatomyositis

469. A 20-year-old man with a family history of asthma and hay fever complains of chronic pruritus. Examination reveals dry, crusted, excoriated lesions of the face and antecubital fossae. The most likely diagnosis is
- **A.** atopic eczema
- **B.** stasis dermatitis
- **C.** seborrheic dermatitis
- **D.** dermatitis herpetiformis
- **E.** lichen planus

470. Skin tags may be an external manifestation of which internal disorder?

A. Colonic polyps
B. Coronary artery disease
C. Diabetes mellitus
D. Diverticulosis
E. Cholelithiasis

471. The finding of numerous spider angiomas in a 40-year-old man suggests the diagnosis of

A. cirrhosis
B. diabetes mellitus
C. a feminizing tumor
D. rheumatoid arthritis
E. thyrotoxicosis

472. Telangiectasias confined to the periungual area suggest the diagnosis of

A. cirrhosis
B. a connective tissue disease
C. a basal cell carcinoma
D. hereditary hemorrhagic telangiectasia
E. actinic keratosis

473. A nodule is noted in a sun-exposed area. Its surface is pearl-like and superficial telangiectasias are present. The most likely diagnosis is

A. a basal cell carcinoma
B. seborrheic keratosis
C. a squamous cell carcinoma
D. a melanoma
E. Bowen's disease

474. Axillary "freckles" are diagnostic of

A. Albright's disease
B. acanthosis nigricans
C. melasma
D. neurofibromatosis
E. senile lentigo

475. A patient presents with abscesses, sinus tracts, and scarring of the axilla. Examination also reveals perianal abscesses. The most likely diagnosis is
A. tuberculosis
B. ulcerative colitis
C. hidradenitis suppurativa
D. actinomycosis
E. furuncles

476. A middle-aged alcoholic patient demonstrates blister formation on sun-exposed areas that frequently ulcerate and ultimately form scars. The most likely diagnosis is
A. pemphigus
B. erythema multiforme
C. poison ivy dermatitis
D. herpes zoster
E. porphyria cutanea tarda

477. "Target" or "iris" lesions strongly suggest the diagnosis of
A. Reiter's disease
B. pemphigus
C. erythema multiforme
D. urticaria
E. Behcet's syndrome

478. Cyanosis is usually clinically apparent when the concentration of unsaturated capillary hemoglobin exceeds
A. 1 g%
B. 2 g%
C. 3 g%
D. 4 g%
E. 5 g%

479. A 45-year-old man develops velvety, brown plaques in the axilla and groin. His weight is normal, and there is no family history of such a problem. No endocrinopathies are present. This patient is likely to develop
A. diabetes mellitus
B. a carcinoma
C. coronary artery disease
D. myasthenia gravis
E. amyloidosis

480. A 52-year-old man undergoes a routine physical examination. A focal area of white scalp hair contrasts with his otherwise brown hair. This abnormality may be seen with all of the following EXCEPT

A. alopecia areata
B. piebaldism
C. vitiligo
D. tuberous sclerosis
E. albinism

481. Rubbing a brownish macule produces a wheal. This is diagnostic of

A. neurofibromatosis
B. tuberous sclerosis
C. Addison's disease
D. fibrous dysplasia
E. urticaria pigmentosa

482. A woman receiving oral contraceptives develops a fever and multiple inflamed nodules on the anterior tibial surfaces. The most likely diagnosis is

A. erythema nodosum
B. thrombophlebitis
C. gonococcemia
D. erysipelas
E. Weber–Christian disease

483. A patient with ulcerative colitis develops a spontaneous large ulcer on the anterior tibia. It is very tender, and its edges are undermined. The most likely diagnosis is

A. venous insufficiency
B. skin carcinoma
C. arterial insufficiency
D. a decubitus ulcer
E. pyoderma gangrenosum

484. A patient complains of a rash and itching. Examination reveals threadlike lesions involving the webs between the fingers and secondary excoriations. The most likely diagnosis is
A. pediculosis
B. a flea bite
C. scabies
D. neurodermatitis
E. eczema

485. Subcutaneous crepitus is pathognomonic for subcutaneous emphysema and
A. degenerative arthritis
B. lipodystrophy
C. tenosynovitis
D. gas gangrene
E. none of the above

486. Perifollicular hyperkeratosis and petechiae suggest the diagnosis of
A. amyloidosis
B. uremia
C. scurvy
D. cryoglobulinemia
E. thrombocytopenia

487. The most common cause of onycholysis is probably
A. hyperthyroidism
B. photosensitivity reactions
C. psoriasis
D. a *Pseudomonas* infection
E. trauma

488. The most useful feature to distinguish an Osler's node from a Janeway lesion is its
A. distribution
B. configuration
C. tenderness on palpation
D. frequency of occurrence
E. association with acute endocarditis

489. Transverse fingernail grooves are known as
- **A.** Mee's lines
- **B.** Beau's lines
- **C.** Terry's nails
- **D.** Lindsay's nails
- **E.** Muehrcke's lines

490. Inflammatory arthritis and pitted fingernails suggest the diagnosis of
- **A.** degenerative arthritis
- **B.** rheumatoid arthritis
- **C.** Reiter's syndrome
- **D.** psoriasis
- **E.** gout

491. Unilateral clubbing and unidigital clubbing of the nails suggest the diagnosis of
- **A.** inflammatory bowel disease
- **B.** a lung abscess
- **C.** bronchiectasis
- **D.** a localized vascular lesion
- **E.** a carcinoma of the lung

492. Spoon nails are most commonly associated with
- **A.** iron deficiency anemia
- **B.** rheumatic fever
- **C.** lichen planus
- **D.** syphilis
- **E.** tuberculosis

493. The single most reliable clinical finding to establish the diagnosis of clubbing is
- **A.** flattening of the angle between the proximal nail plate and the dorsal surface of the distal phalanx
- **B.** greater nail mobility
- **C.** cyanotic discoloration
- **D.** increased nail curvature
- **E.** increased size of the eponychium

494. A 22-year-old woman develops an acute syndrome characterized by fever, hemorrhagic–pustular skin lesions, and monoarticular arthritis. The most likely diagnosis is

A. systemic lupus erythematosus
B. rheumatoid arthritis
C. Reiter's syndrome
D. Henoch–Schönlein purpura
E. gonococcemia

495. A pigmented papule less than 1 cm, which dimples when lateral digital pressure is applied, is probably

A. a melanoma
B. a dermatofibroma
C. a senile keratosis
D. a junctional nevus
E. an intradermal nevus

496. A red, 5-mm, circumscribed lesion is present under a fingernail. It is very painful on palpation. The most likely diagnosis is

A. a fibroma
B. a nevus
C. an angioma
D. a glomus tumor
E. a melanoma

497. Red, nonblanching, 2–3-mm papular lesions found on the trunk of an adult are probably

A. angiokeratomas
B. cherry angiomas
C. petechiae
D. spider telangiectasias
E. hereditary hemorrhagic telangiectasias

498. Diffusely yellow nails are related to

A. fungal infections
B. cirrhosis
C. uremia
D. impaired lymphatic drainage
E. fluorisis

499. A young man presents with recurring attacks of abdominal pain and multiple, 2–5-mm, brown macules on the lips, buccal mucosa, and the dorsum of the fingers. The most likely diagnosis is

A. Addison's disease
B. hereditary hemorrhagic telangiectasia
C. Gardner's syndrome
D. Peutz–Jeghers syndrome
E. a normal variant

500. During a 10-week period a 70-year-old man develops a 3-cm tumor on his left cheek. Its surface is translucent and there is a central keratinous plug. The most likely diagnosis is

A. a cutaneous horn
B. Bowen's disease
C. a basal cell carcinoma
D. a squamous cell carcinoma
E. a keratoacanthoma

501. A patient develops erythematous, scaling plaques at sites of trauma. Characteristic punctate bleeding points are produced by abrading the scale. The most likely diagnosis is

A. seborrheic dermatitis
B. psoriasis
C. lichen planus
D. atopic dermatitis
E. pityriasis rosea

502. The hemoglobin concentration at which the palmar creases first lose their pink color is approximately

A. 13 g/dL
B. 11 g/dL
C. 9 g/dL
D. 7 g/dL
E. 5 g/dL

503. An elderly woman has had a 3-cm, tan, frecklelike lesion for several years. The lesion has grown slowly and multiple areas of increased and decreased pigmentation have appeared. The most likely diagnosis is

A. senile lentigo
B. lentigo maligna melanoma
C. superficial spreading melanoma
D. nodular melanoma
E. lentigo

504. A patient notes a tender spot on the sole of his foot. Examination reveals a central dark core that is very tender when pressed against the adjacent metatarsal head. Tiny dark spots overlie the lesion. The most likely diagnosis is

A. a plantar wart
B. a melanoma
C. a corn
D. an inflamed bursa
E. a callus

505. After tending her grandchildren, a 50-year-old woman develops red facial macules. These lesions subsequently become vesicles that rupture and form yellow "stuck-on" crusts. The most likely diagnosis is

A. varicella
B. acne rosacea
C. contact dermatitis
D. impetigo
E. folliculitis

506. A 32-year-old man develops a pruritic, scaling rash that is most marked on the trunk. The problem was preceded by a 4-cm, red, scaling plaque. The lesions are maculopapular and follow the lines of cleavage of the skin. The most likely diagnosis is

A. lichen planus
B. pityriasis rosea
C. seborrheic dermatitis
D. a drug eruption
E. syphilis

507. A hard, pointed, 10-mm hyperkeratotic lesion has grown slowly on the cheek of an elderly man. This is most likely
A. seborrheic keratosis
B. a keratoacanthoma
C. an acrochordon
D. a cutaneous horn
E. sebaceous hyperplasia

508. A 45-year-old woman presents with diffusely yellow skin and normal appearing sclerae. This is most likely due to
A. jaundice
B. carotenemia
C. antimalarial therapy
D. hemolytic anemia
E. hypothyroidism

509. For several years a 42-year-old man has noted "lumps" on the extremities and trunk. Most of the lesions are discrete and have a lobulated texture. The most likely diagnosis is
A. multiple lipomata
B. multiple sebaceous cysts
C. metastatic carcinoma
D. multiple verrucae
E. multiple keloids

510. Which of the following is a premalignant skin lesion?
A. Seborrheic keratosis
B. An epidermal cyst
C. Actinic keratosis
D. Seborrheic dermatitis
E. Vitiligo

511. Dry, coarse hair suggests the diagnosis of
A. myxedema
B. pituitary insufficiency
C. Grave's disease
D. alopecia areata
E. Parkinson's disease

512. Ossification of the skin or subcutaneous tissue is seen in all of the following EXCEPT
A. scleroderma
B. basal cell carcinoma
C. nevi
D. hypoparathyroidism
E. pseudohypoparathyrodism

513. An acutely ill patient presents with fever and "palpable" (papular) purpura. The differential diagnosis includes all of the following EXCEPT
A. systemic vasculitis
B. septicemia
C. Rocky Mountain spotted fever
D. a consumption coagulopathy
E. platelet abnormalities

514. Hyperpigmentation in scars and creases suggests the diagnosis of
A. Addison's disease
B. hemochromatosis
C. porphyria cutanea tarda
D. malabsorption
E. hepatic failure

515. A 50-year-old man suddenly develops a large number of seborrheic keratoses on the shoulders and extremities. He should be evaluated for
A. a melanoma
B. an immunodeficiency state
C. tuberculosis
D. a gastric carcinoma
E. arsenic poisoning

516. A 76-year-old woman notes flesh-colored papules on the trunk and eyelids. Intracutaneous bleeding develops in these lesions, both spontaneously and after minimal trauma, e.g., rubbing the eyelid. The most likely diagnosis is

A. amyloidosis
B. sarcoidosis
C. lupus erythematosus
D. thrombocytopenia
E. leprosy

517. Tendon xanthomas suggest the diagnosis of type

A. I hyperlipoproteinemia
B. II hyperlipoproteinemia
C. III hyperlipoproteinemia
D. IV hyperlipoproteinemia
E. V hyperlipoproteinemia

DIRECTIONS: Each of the questions or incomplete statements below is followed by five suggested answers or completions. Select either true (T) or false (F) for **each** option given.

---

518. The major determinants of the normal "flesh" skin color are

A. reflection of red rays
B. reflection of brown rays
C. reflection of yellow rays
D. reflection of blue rays
E. scattering of blue rays

519. Characteristics of a pigmented skin lesion that should point to the need for biopsy include

A. a papular appearance
B. variegated colors
C. irregular borders
D. a uniformly brown color
E. an irregular surface

520. A macule is
- **A.** a circumscribed, nonelevated change in skin color
- **B.** a circumscribed, elevated skin lesion
- **C.** characterized by desquamation
- **D.** produced by alterations in either the epidermis or the dermis
- **E.** characterized by either increased or decreased pigmentation

521. Subungual splinter hemorrhages are associated with
- **A.** bacterial endocarditis
- **B.** trauma
- **C.** the normal state
- **D.** trichinosis
- **E.** mitral stenosis

522. Alopecia areata
- **A.** is a diffuse loss of hair
- **B.** is confined to the scalp
- **C.** may be accompanied by nail ridging and pitting
- **D.** is usually accompanied by another skin disorder
- **E.** is commonly associated with an autoimmune disorder

523. Telangiectasias are characteristic of which of the following?
- **A.** Actinically damaged skin
- **B.** Necrobiosis lipoidica
- **C.** Acne rosacea
- **D.** Erythema multiforme
- **E.** Radiation dermatitis

524. The differential diagnosis of nail hypertrophy includes
- **A.** psoriasis
- **B.** vascular insufficiency
- **C.** trauma
- **D.** fungal infections
- **E.** a congenital abnormality

525. A 45-year-old woman complains of recurrent bouts of flushing. The differential diagnosis includes
A. the menopause
B. the carcinoid syndrome
C. systemic mastocytosis
D. medullary carcinoma of the thyroid
E. emotional stimuli

526. Generalized erythematous scaling may be associated with which of the following?
A. A drug reaction
B. A lymphoma
C. Leukemia
D. Psoriasis
E. Atopic dermatitis

527. Patients with vitiligo
A. develop lesions in areas of trauma
B. often demonstrate mucosal depigmentation
C. may experience spontaneous repigmentation
D. are usually asymptomatic
E. demonstrate hypomelanosis of the skin and hair

528. Features of the atypical pigmented nevi seen in the dysplastic nevus syndrome include
A. typically larger than ordinary nevi
B. variegated color
C. irregular borders and surface
D. location in sun-exposed areas
E. location in sun-protected areas

529. A 60-year-old woman has had hyperkeratotic lesions of the palms and soles for several years. As a child she received chronic therapy with Fowler's solution. She is at risk to develop
A. Bowen's disease of the skin
B. a basal cell carcinoma
C. a melanoma
D. a squamous cell carcinoma
E. an internal carcinoma

14 The Vital Signs

DIRECTIONS: Each of the questions or incomplete statements below is followed by five suggested answers or completions. Select the **one** that is best in each case.

530. According to the American Heart Association, the diastolic blood pressure in adults corresponds closely to the

A. first phase of Korotkoff
B. second phase of Korotkoff
C. third phase of Korotkoff
D. fourth phase of Korotkoff
E. fifth phase of Korotkoff

531. The auscultatory gap may result in erroneously

A. high systolic blood pressure determinations
B. low diastolic blood pressure determinations
C. low systolic and diastolic blood pressure determinations
D. high systolic and diastolic blood pressure determinations
E. low systolic or high diastolic blood pressure determinations

532. An obese patient's blood pressure is noted to be elevated using a standard cuff. The next step in this patient's evaluation should be to

A. measure the blood pressure with a larger cuff
B. measure the blood pressure with a smaller cuff
C. recheck the blood pressure with a standard cuff
D. obtain an intraarterial blood pressure determination
E. evaluate the patient for "curable" causes of hypertension

533. When the sounds of Korotkoff in the antecubital fossa are so faint that an accurate blood pressure cannot be obtained, the next step should be to

A. elevate the patient's legs
B. decrease the venous pressure in the forearm and repeat the blood pressure measurement
C. use the "flush" method of obtaining the blood pressure
D. use the "palpatory" method of obtaining the blood pressure
E. obtain an intraarterial blood pressure

534. A normotensive patient's blood pressure is measured in the supine and erect positions. The expected change in blood pressure in the erect position is a slight

A. increase in the systolic and diastolic pressures
B. decrease in the systolic and diastolic pressures
C. increase in the diastolic and slight decrease in the systolic pressure
D. increase in the systolic and a slight decrease in the diastolic pressure
E. increase in the systolic and no change in the diastolic pressure

535. Elderly patients may demonstrate spurious elevation of the systolic blood pressure due to vessel sclerosis. Select the clinical feature that is most predictive of this problem.

A. A diagonal ear lobe crease
B. A wide pulse pressure
C. A palpable brachial artery when the blood pressure cuff is inflated above the systolic pressure
D. Postural hypotension
E. An antecubital fossa bruit

536. The fifth phase of Korotkoff is defined as a
A. muffling of sound
B. cessation of sound
C. swishing sound
D. soft tapping sound
E. sharp tapping sound

537. The pulse pressure is narrowed with
A. a complete heart block
B. hypertension
C. constrictive pericarditis
D. thyrotoxicosis
E. a sinus bradycardia

538. An elderly patient with cerebrovascular disease and congestive heart failure has apneic episodes lasting 20 seconds followed by 30-second cycles of breathing. The latter begin slowly, peak with tachypnea and hyperpnea, and taper off to an apneic cycle. This is
A. hippocratic respiration
B. Biot's respiration
C. periodic respiration
D. stertorous respiration
E. Kussmaul respiration

539. Sighing respirations suggest the diagnosis of
A. chronic obstructive pulmonary disease
B. metabolic acidosis
C. an anxiety reaction
D. a brainstem lesion
E. congestive heart failure

540. When comparing the mercury and the aneroid sphygmomanometers, all of the following favor the former EXCEPT
A. cost
B. accuracy
C. durability
D. size
E. maintenance

541. The normal adult resting respiratory rate should NOT exceed

A. 10 cycles/min
B. 12 cycles/min
C. 14 cycles/min
D. 16 cycles/min
E. 18 cycles/min

542. Select the correct statement about the effect of tachypnea on electronically measured oral temperatures.

A. It increases the rectal–oral temperature difference
B. It decreases the rectal–oral temperature difference
C. It has no effect on the rectal–oral temperature difference
D. It contributes to prompt recognition of fever
E. As tachypnea increases the rectal–oral temperature difference decreases

---

DIRECTIONS: Each of the questions or incomplete statements below is followed by five suggested answers or completions. Select either true (T) or false (F) for **each** option given.

---

543. A pulse deficit may be found with

A. atrial fibrillation
B. trigeminy
C. ventricular premature contractions
D. atrial premature contractions
E. bigeminy

544. When the blood pressure is measured in the thigh

A. it should be taken with the patient in a supine position
B. it should be taken with a 20-cm bag
C. the systolic blood pressure is usually the same as in the arm
D. the diastolic blood pressure is usually 10–30 mm Hg higher than in the arm
E. it should be measured in both legs

545. An elderly patient is brought into an emergency room with a rectal temperature of 28°C. In this setting, which of the following physical findings may be present?

A. Unresponsiveness to stimuli
B. Apparently absent pulses
C. Rigid joints
D. Absent pupillary reflexes
E. Apparently absent respiration

546. "Factitious fever" should be suspected when

A. the pulse and respiratory rate remain normal during febrile episodes
B. there is no diaphoresis after lysis of fever
C. there are temperature spokes above 104°F
D. the patient has multiple organ system problems
E. there is disagreement between the temperature of a freshly voided urine specimen and the rectal temperature

547. Palpation of the radial pulse while pumping up the sphygmomanometer cuff

A. is unnecessary
B. is helpful in correctly identifying the auscultatory gap
C. is indicated only when the sounds of Korotkoff are faint
D. precludes unnecessarily pumping up the cuff too high
E. is helpful in identifying the first phase of Korotkoff by auscultation

548. Which is a correct interpretation of the blood pressure 140/82/0 mm Hg?

A. Phase I/phase II/phase V
B. Systolic BP = 140, diastolic BP = 0
C. Phase I/phase IV/phase V
D. A high output cardiac state may be present
E. The patient should be evaluated for postural hypotension

549. A wide pulse pressure is found in which of the following conditions?

A. Beriberi heart disease
B. A patent ductus arteriosus
C. Aortic insufficiency
D. A peripheral arteriovenous fistula
E. Coarctation of the aorta

550. In an adult a blood pressure difference of more than 20 mm Hg between the arms may be an important clue for the diagnosis of

A. aortic insufficiency
B. arteriosclerotic disease of the subclavian artery
C. the subclavian steal syndrome
D. the thoracic outlet syndrome
E. the Leriche syndrome

Explanatory Answers

The Abdomen

1. (E) When palpating for the liver edge, the examiner should begin just above the right inguinal area and inch upward toward the right costal margin. If this approach is not used, the examiner may not detect an enlarged liver because the examining hand may be above the liver edge. (Ref. 109)

2. (D) The liver edge, different parts of the colon, the right lower pole of the kidney, and the aorta may be normally palpable. A palpable spleen is probably abnormal. (Ref. 114, p. 88)

3. (B) In a study of the patients with possible ascites, flank dullness was the physical sign with the greatest sensitivity. However, in these patients physical signs had a low predictive value, and the use of ultrasonography may be indicated. (Ref. 21)

4. (C) Rebound tenderness is due to involvement of the parietal peritoneum and is a reliable indicator of peritonitis. (Ref. 23, p. 288)

5. (D) Because bilirubin is taken up readily by the elastin-rich tissues of the sclera, slight jaundice may be first detected by examining this site. (Ref. 92, p. 203)

6. (B) The recognition of clinical jaundice is dependent upon several factors. In general, jaundice is noted when the total bilirubin exceeds 2.0–2.5 mg%. (Ref. 92, p. 203)

7. (B) A femoral hernia may be distinguished from an inguinal hernia because the former lies below the inguinal ligament and lateral to the pubic tubercle. (Ref. 23, p. 260)

8. (D) An abscess in the sacrococcygeal area is often due to an infected pilonidal cyst and tract from which tufts of hair may protrude (Ref. 8, p. 301)

9. (D) In the presence of tense ascites, ballottement may be the best technique for detecting hepatosplenomegaly. (Ref. 16, p. 237)

10. (A) In contrast to many causes of severe abdominal pain, the pain of biliary colic is not exacerbated by movement, and the patient often moves restlessly. (Ref. 61, p. 1531)

11. (D) The diagnosis of paralytic ileus cannot be made unless the clinician has demonstrated absent bowel sounds for at least 3 minutes. (Ref. 23, p. 312)

12. (C) Boardlike rigidity of the anterior abdominal wall is an almost constant finding with a perforated peptic ulcer. (Ref. 103, p. 106)

13. (A) The initial pain of appendicitis is usually referred to the epigastric or periumbilical area. This pain may be due to increased appendiceal peristalsis. (Ref. 103, p. 65)

14. (B) In the presence of acute cholecystitis inspiratory arrest may occur, as the inflamed gallbladder descends and contacts the examiner's fingers (Murphy's sign). (Ref. 31, p. 329)

15. (A) The correct sequence of signs and symptoms seen with acute appendicitis is: epigastric pain, nausea or vomiting, local iliac tenderness, and fever. (Ref. 103, p. 71)

16. (D) McBurney's point corresponds to the base of the normally located appendix. Tenderness at this point may be a sign of appendicitis. The point lies about 2 in. from the right anterior superior iliac spine on a line connecting the umbilicus and the spine. (Ref. 23, p. 289)

17. (B) A pulsatile liver is usually due to severe tricuspid insufficiency. (Ref. 28, p. 516)

18. (B) The normal prostate gland is palpable as a firm structure immediately adjacent to the anterior rectal mucosa. It measures about 4 cm in width and 3 cm in height. A median groove is normally palpable. (Ref. 16, p. 289)

19. (D) Auscultation of the abdomen should precede any maneuver, e.g., palpation, which may stimulate bowel sounds. The latter may interfere with assessment of other abdominal sounds. (Ref. 28, p. 497)

20. (E) A diastasis recti is a separation of the rectus abdominis muscles, which appears as a midline abdominal ridge when intra-abdominal pressure is increased. (Ref. 8, p. 250)

21. (C) The diagnosis of internal hemorrhoids is established best by anoscopic examination. (Ref. 120, p. 790)

22. (A) Narrowing of the celiac artery, which is most often due to extrinsic compression, is the most common cause of an epigastric abdominal bruit. (Ref. 78)

23. (B) Heartburn is the characteristic symptom of esophageal reflux, and it may be exacerbated by overeating or lying down. (Ref. 92, p. 1693)

24. (A) A continuous abdominal venous hum is always abnormal and is virtually pathognomonic of portal hypertension. (Ref. 52)

25. (C) The Richter type of hernia is characterized by involvement of only a portion of the bowel circumference, e.g., the side of the small intestine protrudes through the obturator foramen. (Ref. 28, p. 554)

26. (C) Normally, the flow of blood in anterior abdominal wall vessels is away from the umbilicus. When the upper abdominal veins drain downward, the diagnosis of superior vena caval obstruction is suggested. (Ref. 95, p. 307)

27. (C) Approximately 30% of rectal cancers are palpable on digital rectal examination. (Ref. 72, p. 77)

28. (C) The aorta normally bifurcates at the level of the umbilicus; hence, abdominal aortic pulsations noted below this level suggest the diagnosis of an aortic aneurysm. (Ref. 91, p. 89)

29. (C) Retroperitoneal hemorrhage, as is seen with acute pancreatitis and a ruptured aortic aneurysm, may produce flank ecchymoses; this is the Grey–Turner sign. (Ref. 28, p. 479)

30. (D) The transpyloric plane, which lies midway between the umbilicus and the xiphisternal junction, passes through several important structures, e.g., the renal artery, the pancreas, the duodenum, and the transverse colon. (Ref. 7, p. 16)

31. (A) An acute bowel obstruction is usually accompanied by loud rushes of peristaltic activity, i.e., borborygmi. (Ref. 31, p. 334)

32. A. (F)
B. (T)
C. (T)
D. (T)
E. (T)

Several blood dyscrasias are associated with splenomegaly; however, in sickle-cell anemia recurrent splenic infarcts lead to a fibrous remnant which isn't palpable. (Ref. 124, p. 929)

33. A. (F)
B. (T)
C. (F)
D. (F)
E. (T)

Costovertebral angle tenderness is seen with pyelonephritis and a perinephric abscess. (Ref. 28, p. 512)

34. A. (T)
B. (F)
C. (F)
D. (T)
E. (F)

Visible peristalsis is most often seen with subacute intestinal obstruction; it may also be seen in thin, normal individuals. (Ref. 103, p. 152)

35. A. (T) The normal liver height in men, as determined by
B. (F) percussion in the midclavicular line, may be up to 15
C. (T) cm. Percussion results correlate well with liver scan
D. (F) results. The normal limits vary with sex and lean body
E. (F) mass. (Ref. 20)

36. A. (F) An easily palpable liver edge is not synonymous with
B. (T) hepatomegaly; it may indicate downward displace-
C. (T) ment of a normal liver due to, e.g., emphysema, a
D. (F) right-sided pleural effusion, and ptosis of the liver.
E. (T) (Ref. 120, p. 771)

37. A. (T) Visceral pain is poorly localized. Visceral afferent fi-
B. (T) bers are sensitive to smooth muscle distention, in-
C. (T) flammation and ischemia. Visceral pain arising from
D. (T) the stomach, duodenum, gallbladder, and pancreas is
E. (F) usually referred to the epigastrium. (Ref. 53, p. 667)

38. A. (F) A rectal examination in a patient with an uncompli-
B. (T) cated acute myocardial infarction may be safely done
C. (F) and provides important data concerning occult gas-
D. (F) trointestinal bleeding, prostatic enlargement, and
E. (T) whether the patient has a fecal impaction. (Ref. 35)

The Breast

39. (A) Breast cancer is found most often in the upper outer quadrant, which includes the axillary tail. (Ref. 23, p. 168)

40. (C) An eczematous nipple lesion suggests the diagnosis of Paget's disease. It is associated with ductal carcinoma of the underlying breast. (Ref. 112, p. 548)

41. (C) A bloody nipple discharge is most commonly due to a benign intraductal papilloma. Only about 1% of breast cancer patients demonstrate a bloody nipple discharge. (Ref. 95, p. 231)

42. (C) Carcinoma of the male breast is usually found beneath the nipple or areola. (Ref. 50, p. 782)

43. (E) Retraction phenomena suggest the presence of carcinoma of the breast. They are produced by fibrotic changes in the suspensory ligaments of the breast. (Ref. 50, p. 114)

44. (B) The diagnosis of gynecomastia is established by palpating a disk-shaped mass of tissue in the subareolar region. The mass should be at least 2 cm in diameter. Palpation also allows the examiner to distinguish gynecomastia from an enlarged breast due to adipose tissue. (Ref. 124, p. 1400)

45. (E) Acute mastitis is very unusual in the nonlactating breast; its presence suggests the diagnosis of an inflammatory breast carcinoma. (Ref. 50, p. 576)

46. (B) Breast nodularity associated with intermittent tenderness suggests the diagnosis of chronic cystic mastitis; however, with this disorder breast examination is not conclusive, and a biopsy may be necessary to establish a firm diagnosis. (Ref. 92, p. 790)

47. (B) Palpable, asymptomatic gynecomastia may be found in as many as 30% of normal men. (Ref. 19)

48. (E) The combination of the physical examination and mammography is the most effective screening tool for breast cancer. Self-examination also plays an important role in detecting breast cancer. (Ref. 12, p. 1156)

49. (D) The most likely cause for a nontender, well-defined breast "lump" in a young woman is a fibroadenoma; however, a biopsy is indicated to distinguish this from a malignant neoplasm. (Ref. 28, p. 262)

50. A. (F)
B. (F)
C. (T)
D. (T)
E. (T)

Palpatory features of a breast "lump" that suggest a carcinoma include hardness, irregular margins, a single dominant mass, and apparent attachment to surrounding tissue. (Ref. 50, p. 108)

51. A. (T) The inframammary fold, the axillary tail of the breast,
B. (F) and chronic nipple inversion are normal variants that
C. (T) are not associated with carcinoma of the breast. (Ref.
D. (T) 50, p. 104)
E. (F)

52. A. (T) Duct ectasia, traumatic fat necrosis, and a low-grade
B. (T) abscess may all closely simulate a breast carcinoma
C. (T) on physical examination. (Ref. 50, p. 141)
D. (F)
E. (T)

The Chest and Lungs

53. (C) The normal breath sounds heard over most of the lung fields are vesicular. They are low-pitched, rustling sounds heard throughout inspiration and in early expiration. (Ref. 114, p. 181)

54. (E) Pleural fluid impairs transmission of sound waves to the chest wall; hence, diminished breath sounds and decreased tactile fremitus are noted. Unless there is underlying lung disease, rales are not found with a pleural effusion. (Ref. 8, p. 154)

55. (C) Pneumonia with consolidation is characterized by several physical findings including increased fremitus, dullness to percussion, bronchial breath sounds, bronchophony, and pectoriloquy. (Ref. 70, p. 65)

56. (D) When consolidated lung tissue is in contact with a patent bronchus, the transmission of pulmonary vibrations is enhanced. (Ref. 28, p. 319)

57. (A) In emphysematous patients, the heart sounds may be heard best in the epigastrium. (Ref. 14, p. 30)

58. (C) The physical findings anticipated with a pneumothorax include reduced breath sounds, absent tactile fremitus, reduced chest expansion on inspiration, increased resonance to percussion on the involved side, and deviation of the trachea to the involved side. (Ref. 58, p. 269)

59. (B) Rales (crackles) are probably produced by the opening of previously closed small airways. (Ref. 120, p. 636)

60. (D) Both a rhonchus and a pleural friction rub may be heard during inspiration and expiration. (Ref. 8, p. 152)

61. (B) The physical findings of pneumonia may be confined to a very localized area when the right middle lobe is involved. (Ref. 58, p. 265)

62. (C) A stridor is a high-pitched "crowing" sound heard on inspiration. It is associated with narrowing of the glottis. (Ref. 28, p. 175)

63. (E) The relative duration of inspiration and expiration is the single most useful characteristic distinguishing vesicular, bronchovesicular, and bronchial breath sounds. (Ref. 28, p. 308)

64. (C) The oblique fissure separates the upper and lower lobes. It intercepts the vertebral line at T-4 and the midaxillary line at the fifth rib; hence the lower lobes occupy most of the posterior lung fields. (Ref. 95, p. 192)

65. (E) Because there is greater respiratory movement of the lower anterolateral chest wall, asymmetric respiratory excursion can be detected best when the hands are placed at this site. (Ref. 95, p. 199)

66. (A) Intercostal space retraction is seen with several different respiratory problems; the common pathophysiologic mechanism is decreased pulmonary compliance. (Ref. 17, p. 130)

67. (C) Airway obstruction may be documented at the bedside by listening over the trachea while the patient forcibly expires after deep inhalation. A forced expiratory time of 4.0 seconds or greater is abnormal. (Ref. 63, p. 118)

68. (C) Normally, with quiet breathing the inspiratory and expiratory time intervals are equal. With obstructive lung disease the expiratory component lengthens. (Ref. 17, p. 130)

69. (A) A study using time-expanded wave-form analysis demonstrated that rales are discontinuous sounds whereas rhonchi are continuous sounds. (Ref. 84)

70. (A) The wheeze is the characteristic physical finding of asthma; however, there is poor correlation between airway obstruction and wheezing. (Ref. 85)

71. (B) Egophony is heard over areas of consolidation and at the upper margin of pleural effusions. It is a type of bronchophony. As the patient says "E" the auscultator hears an "A" sound over the involved area. (Ref. 95, p. 214)

72. (D) Breathing through pursed lips is seen with obstructive airway disease. This maneuver increases intraluminal airway pressure and helps prevent airway collapse. (Ref. 17, p. 130)

73. (B) The normal percussion note heard over most of the lung during most of the respiratory cycle is resonance. (Ref. 63, p. 121)

74. (E) Auscultation is the most effective tool for comparing the state of bronchial patency in different parts of the bronchopulmonary tree. (Ref. 63, p. 123)

75. (B) After shallow breathing, auscultation may normally reveal a few basilar, end-inspiratory rales. (Ref. 53, p. 346)

76. (A) Low, fixed diaphragms are characteristic of severe emphysema. Diaphragmatic excursion may also be reduced with pleuritis and with splinting secondary to severe pain. (Ref. 58, p. 264)

77. (B) Auscultatory percussion appears to be a sensitive technique for detecting lung infections and masses; using this method, dullness is more readily discerned than with conventional chest percussion. (Ref. 49)

78. (A) A new nomenclature for pulmonary sounds is developing that is based on acoustic characteristics; discontinuous sounds occurring in brief bursts, which were formerly referred to as "rales," should be designated "crackles." (Ref. 85)

79. (A) A fixed, monophonic wheeze is generated by the passage of a jet of air through an incompletely occluded bronchus. The musical sound is generated by the vibrations of the bronchial walls and tissues producing the narrowing. (Ref. 42, p. 48)

80. (E) Current evidence suggests that normal vesicular breath sounds arise from turbulent flow in lobar and segmental bronchi. (Ref. 70, p. 64)

81. (A) Pulmonary arteriovenous fistulas are an important feature of hereditary hemorrhagic telangiectasia. (Ref. 9, p. 126)

82. (D) Expiration normally occurs passively as a result of the elastic recoil of the lung. In the presence of airway obstruction, the abdominal muscles may function as accessory muscles of expiration. (Ref. 73, p. 166)

83. (D) End-expiratory coughing expels air from hypoventilated areas. Inflation of these areas produces the rales that may be an early clue to the diagnosis of pulmonary tuberculosis. (Ref. 95, p. 217)

84. (A) Kyphoscoliosis can lead to cor pulmonale; patients with this disorder have normal airway resistance in relation to their lung volumes. (Ref. 92, p. 1588)

85. (C) Crackles (rales) that occur early in inspiration are characteristic of patients with severe obstructive lung disease; crackles (rales) that occur in late inspiration are characteristic of patients with restrictive lung disease. (Ref. 70, p. 88)

86. A. (T)
B. (F)
C. (T)
D. (T)
E. (F)

Rhonchi are continuous sounds that are heard in both inspiration and expiration. They are produced by airway narrowing. (Ref. 95, p. 217)

87. A. (F)
B. (F)
C. (T)
D. (T)
E. (T)

Labored respiration is suggested by intercostal retractions, use of the accessory muscles of expiration, and an excessively prolonged expiratory phase. (Ref. 33, p. 15)

88. **A. (F)** **B. (T)** **C. (T)** **D. (F)** **E. (T)**
Bronchial breath sounds are higher pitched, have a longer expiratory phase, and are usually louder than vesicular breath sounds. They are not normally heard over the chest except over the manubrium. (Ref. 33, p. 44)

89. **A. (F)** **B. (T)** **C. (T)** **D. (T)** **E. (T)**
A unilateral decrease in chest expansion may be seen with several disorders, including rib fracture, pleural effusion, pneumonia, and phrenic nerve palsy. (Ref. 33, p. 16)

90. **A. (F)** **B. (T)** **C. (F)** **D. (T)** **E. (T)**
Vocal fremitus, which may also be called tactile fremitus, is due to the transmission of laryngeal vibrations to the chest wall. It is most marked near major airways and is increased with pulmonary consolidation. (Ref. 95, p. 199)

91. **A. (F)** **B. (T)** **C. (F)** **D. (T)** **E. (T)**
The articulation of the second rib with the sternomanubrial junction (angle of Louis) is an important anterior thoracic landmark. (Ref. 95, p. 192)

The Ears, Nose, and Throat

92. (C) Successful otoscopic examination is facilitated by inspecting the external canal before introducing the speculum, choosing the largest speculum that will comfortably fit into the external canal, straightening the external canal by pulling the pinna upwards and backwards, guarding against sudden patient movement, and adjusting the line of vision to allow observation of the entire canal and tympanic membrane. (Ref. 121, p. 18)

93. (E) Movement of the tragus or pinna accentuates the pain of otitis externa; in otitis media with drainage this maneuver is not painful. (Ref. 100, p. 32)

94. (B) An acoustic neuroma is a benign tumor that may be locally destructive. It typically produces a unilateral, progressive, nonfluctuating, neurosensory hearing loss, unilateral tinnitus, and unsteadiness. (Ref. 37, p. 235)

95. (C) Aspirin, other analgesics, and artificial food coloring may produce severe asthmatic attacks in patients with chronic asthma and nasal polyps; sodium salicylate has not been implicated in this disorder. (Ref. 96)

96. (B) The 256 cycles/sec tuning fork is preferred for performing the Weber test. With higher-pitched tuning forks, low-tone deficits may be missed; lower-pitched tuning forks produce excessive vibratory stimulation. (Ref. 120, p. 932)

97. (D) A pigmented metabolite deposited in the connective tissue of patients with alkaptonuria causes the nose and ears to appear blue. Under the microscope the pigment is an ocher color (yellow-orange). (Ref. 38, p. 1049)

98. (A) If the eustachian tube is obstructed, a vacuum is created in the middle ear that results in retraction of the tympanic membrane. (Ref. 100, p. 45)

99. (D) Bullous myringitis is characterized by hemorrhagic vesicles involving the tympanic membranes. It is caused by both *Mycoplasma pneumoniae* and viruses. The former may be successfully treated with erythromycin or tetracycline. (Ref. 82, p. 366)

100. (B) A "hairy" tongue is seen when filiform papillae lengthen abnormally. These papillae may assume a variety of colors due to staining. The condition is benign and symptomless. (Ref. 92, p. 184)

101. (C) Torus palatinus, a midline bony exostosis of the hard palate, is of no clinical significance except in patients who must be fitted with upper dentures. (Ref. 28, p. 167)

102. (A) Leukoplakia is a whitish, indurated lesion of the oral mucosa that is premalignant. Biopsy is necessary to establish the diagnosis. (Ref. 92, p. 186)

103. (D) A "geographic" tongue is an asymptomatic, benign condition of unknown cause. Normal fungiform papillae together with migratory atrophy of the filiform papillae account for the appearance. (Ref. 92, p. 187)

104. (C) Patients with anaerobic pulmonary infections often have a characteristic putrid odor of the breath. (Ref. 31, p. 157)

105. (A) Gingival hypertrophy is associated with puberty, pregnancy, diphenylhydantoin therapy, and leukemia. (Ref. 8, p. 120)

106. (C) The lip is the most common site for oral carcinoma. (Ref. 120, p. 594)

107. (D) Focal sinus tenderness is not specific for acute sinusitis. Visualization of pus draining from a sinus ostium, aspiration of pus from a sinus, and x-ray findings establish a definitive diagnosis. (Ref. 37, p. 275)

108. (B) Cheek swelling is usually due to an apical dental abscess and is only rarely caused by maxillary sinusitis (Ref. 108)

109. (C) Although the appearance of the tympanic membrane may suggest the diagnosis of serous otitis, the diagnosis depends upon demonstrating tympanic membrane immobility with a pneumatic otoscope. (Ref. 37, p. 159)

110. (E) Fluorosis is seen when children drink water containing more than 2 ppm of fluoride. Although the teeth are resistant to caries, they often appear pitted and mottled. (Ref. 125, p. 196)

111. (C) Buccal mucosal sebaceous glands appear as pinhead-sized yellow spots; they are a normal finding. (Ref. 95, p. 168)

112. (C) A rhinophyma is a slowly progressive, bulbous nasal deformity due to hyperplasia of sebaceous glands. It is a manifestation of acne rosacea. (Ref. 37, p. 288)

113. (C) Painless, hard, white deposits along the helix of the ear may be the first clue pointing to the diagnosis of gout; the gouty tophus consists of sodium urate crystals. (Ref. 28, p. 187)

114. (D) Large, orange tonsils are seen in Tangier disease, an unusual disorder associated with decreased levels of high-density lipoprotein. (Ref. 60, p. 131)

115. (D) The rapid development of fever, a sore throat, croup, and drooling suggest the diagnosis of acute epiglottitis. Acute airway obstruction is a life-threatening complication of this disorder. (Ref. 92, p. 1572)

116. (E) "Hairy" leukoplakia is a new form of oral leukoplakia characterized by white plaques on the lateral tongue margins. Numerous projections result in the "hairy" appearance. This lesion has been seen in male homosexuals who are at high risk to develop the acquired immunodeficiency syndrome. (Ref. 48)

117. (B) A healthy tympanic membrane is usually a pearly gray color; other colors are seen in a variety of pathologic conditions, e.g., a blue color with hemotympanium. (Ref. 95, p. 156)

118. (C) A cholesteatoma results from benign proliferation of squamous epithelium. It usually appears as a white nodular lesion near the annulus of the tympanic membrane. It may be locally destructive. (Ref. 17, p. 90)

119. (D) Numerous fragile telangiectasia are part of the hereditary disorder, Osler–Weber–Rendu disease (hereditary hemorrhagic telangiectasia). Spontaneous bleeding from the nose and gastrointestinal tract occurs frequently. (Ref. 92, p. 1900)

120. A. (T) In the modern era, assessment of auditory acuity with the tuning fork remains an important tool. (Ref. 32, p. 298)
B. (F)
C. (T)
D. (F)
E. (T)

121. A. (T) Glossitis is associated with many causes, including iron deficiency, vitamin deficiencies, and the presence of dentures. (Ref. 120, p. 597)
B. (T)
C. (F)
D. (T)
E. (F)

122. A. (T) Multiple neuromas of the tongue have been seen with neurofibromatosis and with the multiple en-
B. (F)

C. (T) docrine adenomatosis syndrome. (Ref. 38, p. 880)
D. (F)
E. (F)

123. **A. (F)** Tonsilar exudate, tender anterior cervical adeno-
B. (F) pathy, and enlarged tonsils are all predictive of a
C. (T) throat culture positive for group A streptococci.
D. (T) (Ref. 67)
E. (T)

The Eye

124. (E) Successful ophthalmoscopic examination is facilitated by using the right eye and hand to examine the right eye, using the left eye and hand to examine the left eye, holding the patient's upper eyelid with the thumb, dimming ambient light, and asking the patient to look straight ahead at a distant object. (Ref. 121, p. 6)

125. (B) Angioid streaks and "plucked chicken" skin are seen in pseudoxanthoma elasticum, which is also characterized by premature arterial vascular disease and gastrointestinal bleeding. (Ref. 92, p. 577)

126. (B) The Marcus Gunn pupil dilates instead of constricting as a light is swung from the normal eye to the eye with an optic nerve or retinal lesion. (Ref. 1, p. 155)

127. (B) The near reflex contributes to near vision by allowing passage of predominantly direct light rays that focus on the retina. This is accomplished by convergence of the visual axes, pupillary constriction, and lens accomodation. (Ref. 119, p. 215)

128. (B) The essential abnormality of hypertensive retinopathy is arteriolar constriction, both focal and generalized. Chronic hypertensive retinopathy contributes to the development of arteriolar sclerosis; widening of the arteriolar light reflex and arteriovenous nicking are signs of arteriolar sclerosis. (Ref. 54, p. 112)

129. (E) Subconjunctival hemorrhage is usually an innocuous event, which is unrelated to other medical problems. Because spontaneous resolution usually occurs, elaborate diagnostic studies should be deferred. (Ref. 8, p. 98)

130. (D) Ocular trauma may result in sudden visual loss due to anterior chamber hemorrhage. This is a hyphema. A blood level may be noted or blood may fill the entire anterior chamber. (Ref. 82, p. 388)

131. (B) Pigmented corneal rings have been observed with the slit lamp in three patients with primary biliary cirrhosis and in one patient with chronic active hepatitis. (Ref. 41)

132. (C) The characteristic visual field defect seen with a pituitary tumor is a bitemporal hemianopsia. (Ref. 1, p. 154)

133. (A) A visual acuity of 20/30 means that the patient sees figures at 20 feet that are normally seen from 30 feet. (Ref. 54, p. 29)

134. (D) Drusen are degenerative hyaline deposits of the elastic membrane separating the retina and choroid. They do not indicate a systemic disease and are usually benign. (Ref. 8, p. 108)

135. (B) The blood in a preretinal hemorrhage characteristically settles out producing the flat-topped appearance. Spontaneous preretinal hemorrhage suggests a blood dyscrasia. (Ref. 54, p. 133)

136. (E) Benign choroidal nevi are not elevated. Elevation of a lesion is a necessary requisite for the diagnosis of a malignant choroidal melanoma. (Ref. 54, p. 154)

137. (A) Pulsations of the retinal veins are visible at the disk in most normal eyes. (Ref. 54, p. 59)

138. (E) The history of the sudden appearance of unilateral "floaters" followed by a peripheral visual field defect strongly suggests the diagnosis of a retinal detachment. Confirmatory ophthalmoscopic findings include an elevated retina and concealment of retinal pigment and choroidal vessels by subretinal fluid. (Ref. 54, p. 390)

139. (D) The optic disk circulation is separate from that of the retina. Pallor of the disk and absence of small peripheral disk vessels strongly suggest the diagnosis of optic atrophy. (Ref. 54, p. 67)

140. (C) The most common cause of unilateral exophthalmos is thyroid ophthalmopathy. It usually progresses to bilateral involvement. (Ref. 54, p. 204)

141. (B) A corneal arcus is a white ring near the limbus. It is an independent risk factor for coronary artery disease in men under 50 years of age. (Ref. 99)

142. (C) Chemosis is conjunctival edema, which in severe cases may appear as a bizarre protrusion between the eyelids. (Ref. 25, p. 9)

143. (E) Intraocular pressure greater than 22 mm Hg may be associated with the development of glaucoma. (Ref. 63, p. 71)

144. (A) Cotton-wool spots are small areas of infarcted nerve fibers due to arteriolar occlusion. (Ref. 25, p. 44)

145. (E) Anisocoria is found as a normal variant in 5% of the population; hence, a patient without other evidence for dysfunction should simply be clinically monitored. (Ref. 54, p. 43)

146. (C) Patients with moderately elevated intraocular pressure and normal visual fields are considered "glaucoma suspects." A large physiologic cup-to-optic-disk ratio is the risk factor most predictive of the subsequent development of glaucoma. (Ref. 62)

147. (D) An ectropion is an outward drooping of the eyelid that causes epiphora, a tearing down the cheek. (Ref. 54, p. 453)

148. (B) Patients with farsightedness (hyperopia) may demonstrate the following ophthalmoscopic findings: a small optic disk, an unusually pink optic disk, small retinal vessels, and an absent optic cup. A "plus" lens is required to visualize the fundus. (Ref. 73, p. 414)

149. (A) A chronic granuloma of the eyelid is due to sterile inflammation of a meibomian (sebaceous) gland. (Ref. 119, p. 44)

150. (C) A pterygium is a fleshy excrescence that extends onto the cornea from the conjunctiva. If vision is impaired, it should be excised. (Ref. 119, p. 82)

151. (C) Osteogenesis imperfecta is a rare hereditary disorder characterized by multiple fractures and blue sclerae; the latter occurs because the sclera is thin and the underlying choroid becomes visible. (Ref. 92, p. 576)

152. (E) When fluorescein staining of the cornea reveals a dendritic ulcer, the diagnosis of an infection with herpes simplex is suggested. (Ref. 54, p. 443)

153. (E) A patient is considered legally blind when the best corrected vision is 20/200 or less in the better eye. (Ref. 54, p. 567)

154. (C) Neovascularization is the essential feature of proliferative diabetic retinopathy. (Ref. 90)

155. (E) Muscae volitantes or "floaters" appear as small, motile dark flecks on ophthalmoscopic examination. They are due to degenerative changes of the vitreous. (Ref. 89, p. 17)

156. (E) Central retinal artery occlusion may present as a sudden loss of vision in one eye. Ophthalmoscopic examination reveals pallor of the fundus and a cherry-red-appearing macula. (Ref. 89, p. 43)

157. (D) Inflammation of the lacrimal gland (dacryoadenitis) is usually confined within the lateral margin of the orbit. (Ref. 28, p. 105)

158. (D) Iritis is characterized by cells in the anterior chamber; these are visualized best with the slit lamp. (Ref. 86, p. 262)

159. (A) The most light-sensitive part of the retina, the macula, should be examined last. (Ref. 31, p. 168)

160. (A) Hypertelorism is seen with several syndromes, e.g., cleidocranial dysostosis. Normally, the distance between the two medial canthi is about one-third the distance between the two lateral canthi; if the medial canthal distance is increased, hypertelorism is present. (Ref. 34, p. 270)

161. (D) Keratitis, iritis, and acute glaucoma are the causes of a red eye that may produce serious ocular damage; circumcorneal or ciliary injection are seen in all of these disorders. (Ref. 22, p. 66)

162. (D) Band keratopathy is the interpalpebral corneal deposition of calcium salts. This is seen with degenerative, inflammatory, and metabolic conditions including various causes of hypercalcemia. (Ref. 119, p. 99)

163. (E) Yellowish eyelid plaques are xanthelasma; they may be associated with hyperlipidemia. (Ref. 95, p. 81)

164. (B) Eversion of the upper eyelid is especially helpful in evaluating the patient with an ocular foreign body. (Ref. 95, p. 104)

165. (C) The dry-eye syndrome is due to many different causes, including aging. The simplest screening test for tear production is the Schirmer test; in this test filter paper is placed in the conjunctival sac, and then wetting of the paper is measured. (Ref. 119, p. 53)

166. (B) With normal ambient light, the normal range of pupillary diameter is 2–6 mm. (Ref. 118, p. 21)

167. (B) Lipemia retinalis is a striking ophthalmoscopic finding in which the fundus appears pale and the vessels appear cream-colored. This is due to hyperlipidemia and is seen with poorly controlled diabetes mellitus. (Ref. 86, p. 445)

168. **A. (F)** **B. (T)** **C. (F)** **D. (T)** **E. (F)**

Nonparalytic strabismus is not associated with diplopia or headaches. If the condition is not recognized and treated, suppression ambylopia develops. (Ref. 54, p. 355)

169. A. (T) When using the ophthalmoscope, corneal light reflection may be minimized by directing the beam of light toward the edge of the pupil, using the small aperture, and using a dust cover/polarizing filter. (Ref. 121, p. 7)
B. (F)
C. (T)
D. (F)
E. (T)

170. A. (F) Several systemic diseases are associated with bilateral cataracts, e.g., hypoparathyroidism, Down's syndrome, galactosemia, and atopic dermatitis. (Ref. 119, p. 126)
B. (T)
C. (F)
D. (T)
E. (T)

171. A. (F) Central retinal vein occlusion results in painless, sudden, unilateral loss of vision. The characteristic appearance includes papilledema, retinal hemorrhages, cotton-wool spots, and venous engorgement. (Ref. 119, p. 139)
B. (T)
C. (T)
D. (T)
E. (F)

172. A. (F) Hard retinal exudates are produced by the intraretinal deposition of lipoids in chronic vascular disorders. They are smaller and have more discrete borders than cotton-wool spots. (Ref. 54, p. 82)
B. (T)
C. (T)
D. (T)
E. (F)

173. A. (T) Early ophthalmoscopic findings of papilledema include blurring of the optic nerve margins, retinal vein distention, loss of retinal vein pulsations, and hyperemia of the optic nerve. (Ref. 74)
B. (F)
C. (T)
D. (F)
E. (T)

174. A. (T) Although the optic disk normally measures only 1.5 mm in diameter, it appears much larger because of the magnifying effect of the lens and cornea. The temporal margin is usually more clearly defined than the nasal margin. (Ref. 95, p. 120)
B. (F)
C. (F)
D. (F)
E. (F)

175. A. (F) Intraretinal hemorrhage assumes a linear, flame-shaped configuration in the superficial nerve fiber layer and a more discrete "dot and blot" configu-
B. (T)
C. (T)

D. (F) ration in the deeper retinal layers. (Ref. 95, p. 128)
E. (T)

176. A. (F) Identification of the macula is important because it
B. (F) contains the only cells specialized for detail vision.
C. (T) It is located temporal to the disk and recognized by
D. (F) its central depression and darker color. (Ref. 54,
E. (T) p. 59)

177. A. (F) A Roth spot is a small hemorrhagic retinal lesion
B. (F) with a central area of pallor; it occurs with endo-
C. (T) carditis and leukemia. (Ref. 28, p. 123)
D. (T)
E. (F)

178. A. (F) The optic nerve does not contain rods and cones. It
B. (T) accounts for the physiologic blind spot that is usually
C. (T) elliptical in shape and located lateral to the point of
D. (F) fixation. (Ref. 29, p. 107)
E. (F)

179. A. (T) Retinal microaneurysms appear as tiny red dots with
B. (T) discrete margins. They are due to capillary dilatation
C. (F) and are seen with diabetes mellitus and retinal
D. (F) branch vein occlusion. (Ref. 54, p. 70)
E. (F)

180. A. (T) Hypertensive retinal abnormalities that are poten-
B. (F) tially reversible include hemorrhages, exudates, and
C. (T) papilledema. The changes of retinal arteriolar scle-
D. (T) rosis are not reversible. (Ref. 92, p. 1479)
E. (F)

181. A. (F) When the eye is turned nasally, the superior oblique
B. (F) is an efficient depressor and the inferior oblique is
C. (T) an efficient elevator. When the eye is turned tem-
D. (F) porally, the superior rectus is an efficient elevator
E. (T) and the inferior rectus is an efficient depressor. (Ref.
75, p. 92)

182. A. (F) Senile macular degeneration is a hereditary disorder
B. (T) that causes slowly progressive loss of central vision.
C. (T) Ophthalmoscopic abnormalities are variable and in-
D. (F) clude hyperpigmentation, hypopigmentation, hem-
E. (T) orrhages, exudates, and macular "holes." (Ref. 54, p. 179)

183. A. (T) Ophthalmoscopic minus lenses neutralize myopia.
B. (F) The slit beam of light aids in assessing retinal con-
C. (T) cavity or convexity. Red-free light is useful in dis-
D. (T) tinguishing retinal melanin from hemoglobin. (Ref.
E. (T) 89, p. 9)

General Appearance and Diseases

184. (E) Bilateral internuclear ophthalmoplegia in a young person strongly suggests the diagnosis of multiple sclerosis. (Ref. 92, p. 2100)

185. (D) Tuberous sclerosis is a phakomatosis (neurologic disorder with congenital abnormalities of the eyes and skin) characterized by mental retardation, a seizure disorder, and adenoma sebaceum. (Ref. 92, p. 2135)

186. (B) The diagnosis of the acquired immunodeficiency syndrome is based on clinical criteria. Patients with this disorder must have either Kaposi's sarcoma or an opportunistic infection. The former may present as rapidly developing, red-purple macules and papules involving the skin and other organs. (Ref. 124, p. 1861)

187. (C) A patient with pellagra (tryptophan–nicotinic acid deficiency) may present with multiple physical findings, including dementia, dermatitis, glossitis, and neuropathy. (Ref. 92, p. 462)

188. (D) Erythromelalgia is a syndrome characterized by burning discomfort of the toes and fingers, which is exacerbated by heat and promptly relieved by aspirin. In patients with thrombocythemia, platelets may mediate inflammatory and occlusive arteriolar changes that produce the syndrome. (Ref. 80)

189. (E) A malnourished patient with confusion, bilateral sixth nerve palsies, horizontal nystagmus, and gait ataxia has the Wernicke–Korsakoff syndrome and should be treated as a medical emergency with intravenous thiamine. (Ref. 92, p. 2113)

190. (C) The nail–patella syndrome is an autosomal dominant disorder characterized by nail dystrophy, absent patellae, accessory iliac horns, and chronic renal disease. Characteristic renal electron microscopic findings are found in all patients with skeletal abnormalities. (Ref. 110, p. 786)

191. (D) Turner's syndrome, gonadal dysgenesis, is characterized by the presence of only one X chromosome in all cells. Unusual physical findings seen with this disorder include a short stature, neck webbing, and sexual infantilism. (Ref. 92, p. 728)

192. (D) Because the physical findings of acromegaly are so characteristic, the diagnosis can often be made accurately at the bedside. Typical features include prominence of the jaw, coarse facial features, a husky voice, and large hands. (Ref. 92, p. 601)

193. (C) A patient with multiple facial cysts and an osteoma of the jaw should be evaluated for Gardner's syndrome. The multiple colonic polyps seen with this syndrome undergo malignant degeneration. (Ref. 38, p. 881)

194. (D) The "slipping rib syndrome" is a disorder of unknown cause that may present as chronic abdominal or chest pain. The diagnosis is established at the bedside by reproducing the pain with the "hooking maneuver." (Ref. 56)

195. (D) Osteitis pubis is an inflammatory disorder of the pubic symphysis. It may occur following surgery or with generalized inflammatory processes, but it may also occur as an idiopathic process. Point tenderness on palpation helps confirm the diagnosis. Treatment with antiinflammatory agents is often very helpful. (Ref. 94, p. 180)

196. (B) Bilateral interruption of corticobulbar fibers to the bulbar nuclei produces the syndrome of pseudobulbar palsy. This is characterized by dysarthria, dysphagia, and emotional lability. (Ref. 29, p. 264)

197. (E) Herpes zoster presents with malaise, pain, and fever that may precede the characteristic unilateral vesicular rash by 2–4 days. (Ref. 124, p. 1723)

198. (B) Polycystic kidney disease may present as palpable right and left upper quadrant masses in a uremic adult. Cystic disease of the kidney may also involve the liver, spleen, and pancreas. (Ref. 92, p. 1666)

199. (A) The toxic shock syndrome has been observed most commonly in women who use tampons. It is due to a staphlococcal infection. A toxin is released that causes diffuse capillary leakage and hypotension. The latter feature distinguishes this disorder from the scalded skin syndrome, the Kawasaki syndrome, and scarlet fever. (Ref. 116)

200. (D) Erysipelas is a superficial streptococcal cellulitis that often presents acutely as a raised, tender area of erythema involving the face and head. (Ref. 38, p. 1430)

201. (C) Reiter's syndrome includes the tetrad of conjunctivitis, urethritis, arthritis, and mucocutaneous lesions, e.g., keratoderma blennorrhagica. (Ref. 92, p. 1989)

202. (D) Fabry's disease is a rare glycolipid storage disorder with characteristic historical and physical findings. The latter include red angiokeratomas, corneal opacities, and spokelike cataracts. (Ref. 38, p. 1128)

203. (C) In chronic renal failure, accumulation of a urochrome together with anemia gives the skin a sallow, yellow appearance. (Ref. 92, p. 1618)

204. (B) The achondroplastic dwarf has a characteristic appearance with a normal trunk, short limbs, a prominent lumbar lordosis, a large head, and a saddle nose. (Ref. 92, p. 1970)

205. (D) Trigeminal neuralgia is characterized by intense bouts of brief, recurrent lancinating pain; the distribution of the pain is usually in the mandibular or maxillary branches of the fifth cranial nerve. The diagnosis is established by the history. (Ref. 92, p. 2152)

206. (D) Splenomegaly is present in more than 75% of patients with polycythemia vera and is the most useful physical finding to distinguish primary from secondary polycythemia. (Ref. 123, p. 1599)

207. (B) When a teenager presents with a fever and sore throat, the occurrence of generalized lymphadenopathy, splenomegaly, and palatal petechiae provide confirmatory evidence for the diagnosis of infectious mononucleosis. (Ref. 12, p. 48)

208. (D) Patients with the Klippel–Feil syndrome are identified because of their short, broad necks; a reduced number of cervical vertebrae and/or fusion of cervical vertebrae account for this unusual configuration. (Ref. 91, p. 17)

209. (D) Temporal arteritis should be strongly suspected when tender, indurated scalp arteries are palpated. Prompt diagnosis and treatment are important to prevent sudden loss of vision. (Ref. 118, p. 17)

210. (E) Adie's syndrome is a rather common cause of asymptomatic anisocoria. The enlarged pupil reacts slowly to light and may accomodate slowly; deep tendon reflexes may also be absent. (Ref. 25, p. 134)

211. A. (F)
B. (T)
C. (F)
D. (T)
E. (F)

Typical features of an adult with prepubertal eunuchoidism include an increased height, an arm span greater than the height, a lower body segment longer than the upper body segment, sparse pubic hair, and a juvenile voice. (Ref. 122, p. 276)

212. A. (T)
B. (F)
C. (F)
D. (T)
E. (T)

The following physical findings suggest the diagnosis of virilization: deepening of the voice, clitoral hypertrophy, and breast atrophy. (Ref. 11, p. 467)

213. A. (T)
B. (T)
C. (F)
D. (T)
E. (T)

The physical examination is especially valuable for assessing vital signs, the general appearance, the severity of illness, visible and palpable lesions, auscultatory abnormalities, respiratory disease, and neurologic dysfunction. (Ref. 53, p. 16)

214. A. (F) The facial appearance of patients with certain diseases, e.g., Parkinson's disease, Cushing's syndrome, Graves' disease, and hypothyroidism, often suggests a specific diagnosis. (Ref. 95, p. 76)
B. (T)
C. (T)
D. (T)
E. (T)

215. A. (T) Characteristic clinical features of an adult with Down's syndrome include a small stature, a large tongue, short fifth fingers, spotty depigmentation of the iris (Brushfield's spots), and a single transverse palmar crease, bilaterally. (Ref. 92, p. 2141)
B. (F)
C. (F)
D. (T)
E. (T)

The Genitalia

216. (C) A varicocele is less apparent in the supine position due to emptying of the dilated pampiniform plexus. A right-sided varicocele is distinctly unusual. (Ref. 23, p. 370)

217. (E) Early carcinoma of the posterior lobe of the prostate is suggested by focal induration. (Ref. 23, p. 359)

218. (B) Nabothian cysts or follicles are commonly seen on speculum examination of the cervix. They are benign lesions that develop when squamous epithelium overgrows columnar epithelium. (Ref. 31, p. 368)

219. (A) With *Trichomonas* vaginitis, the cervix has a characteristic "strawberry" appearance, and the discharge is greenish, profuse, and bubbly; however, the diagnosis is established with a wet mount. (Ref. 120, p. 266)

220. (E) A hard, painless testicular mass is most likely a carcinoma of the testicle. (Ref. 8, p. 269)

221. (A) Bulging of the distal posterior vaginal wall into the introitus is a rectocele; this is demonstrated most readily when the patient bears down. (Ref. 28, p. 630)

222. (E) The syphilitic chancre is characteristically indurated and painless; the diagnosis is established by dark-field examination. (Ref. 31, p. 380)

223. (A) A spermatocele is usually located in the epididymis. (Ref. 28, p. 608)

224. (E) Seventy-five percent of all prostatic carcinomas begin in the posterior lobe. This site is palpable on digital examination of the gland. (Ref. 95, p. 342)

225. (D) In young men with the acute onset of testicular pain, testicular torsion must be correctly diagnosed in order to avoid loss of the testicle. Nuclear scans are the most accurate diagnostic tool for this problem. Emergency surgery may be necessary when a nuclear scan cannot be promptly obtained. (Ref. 55)

226. (B) Reifenstein's syndrome is a form of male pseudohermaphroditism characterized by hypospadias, small testicles, and, often, gynecomastia. (Ref. 122, p. 378)

227. (D) Peyronie's disease is characterized by an area of fibrosis of undetermined cause developing along the shaft of the penis. The area is palpable as a raised plaque. With erection, a chordee is often present. (Ref. 106, p. 546)

228. (B) A moist, verrucous growth on the glans penis suggests the diagnosis of condyloma acuminatum. This viral-induced disorder has a more pointed appearance then the sessile lesions of secondary syphilis. (Ref. 28, p. 598)

229. (D) Sebaceous cysts are common scrotal wall masses. They appear as multiple 5–10-mm yellow cysts. (Ref. 8, p. 269)

230. (C) A persistent, painful erection is a priapism. This may be seen in sickle-cell disease due to vasoocclusion within the corpus cavernosum. Also, it may be seen with other blood dyscrasias, inflammatory and infectious processes, and after prolonged sexual activity. (Ref. 124, p. 929)

231. (B) In the presence of irregular vaginal bleeding, pelvic pain, and unilateral "fullness" of an oviduct, the diagnosis of an ectopic pregnancy must be excluded. (Ref. 28, p. 633)

232. (A) Herpes simplex infection of the genitalia is a venereal disease that, in women, is the most common cause of genital vesicles and ulcers. (Ref. 92, p. 1165)

233. (C) In the presence of pelvic peritonitis, movement of the cervix causes exquisite pain. (Ref. 95, p. 353)

234. (C) A phimosis is present when the prepuce cannot be retracted over the glans penis. (Ref. 28, p. 597)

235. (D) Postmenopausal bleeding is ominous and should be aggressively evaluated with curettage to rule out cancer. (Ref. 92, p. 719)

236. (A) The digital rectal examination is the most sensitive screening tool for prostatic cancer. (Ref. 66)

237. (D) If bowel sounds are auscultated over a scrotal mass, the diagnosis of a scrotal hernia is established. (Ref. 28, p. 604)

238. (B) The labium majora is the anatomic counterpart of the scrotum; hence, women who develop an inguinal hernia may present with groin pain and bulging of the labium. (Ref. 5, p. 965)

239. A. (T)
B. (F)
C. (T)
D. (F)
E. (T)

Normally, the oviduct is difficult to palpate. Normal, approximate dimensions of the female genitalia are as follows: clitoris 1.5 cm in length, cervical os 3–5 mm, uterus 8 cm in length, and ovary 3 cm in length. (Ref. 31, p. 358)

240. A. (F)
B. (F)
C. (T)
D. (T)
E. (F)

The normal mean length of the testicle is 4.5 cm and the normal mean width of the testicle is 2.5 cm. The left testicle normally hangs lower than the right testicle. (Ref. 11, p. 519)

241. A. (F) Uterine physical findings suggestive of the diagnosis
B. (T) of fibroids include nodular enlargement, a firm tex-
C. (T) ture, and mobility. (Ref. 114, p. 117)
D. (F)
E. (T)

242. A. (F) Bluish discoloration of the uterine cervix (Chad-
B. (T) wick's sign) may be seen with pregnancy, congestive
C. (T) heart failure, pelvic tumors, and in women taking
D. (T) oral contraceptives. (Ref. 28, p. 626)
E. (F)

243. A. (T) A fixed, immobile cervix is seen with carcinoma,
B. (T) endometriosis, and pelvic inflammatory disease.
C. (F) Normally, the cervix can be moved 2–3 cm in any
D. (F) direction. (Ref. 95, p. 354)
E. (T)

244. A. (T) Young women with prenatal exposure to diethyl-
B. (F) stilbestrol have a significantly greater incidence of
C. (T) transverse vaginal ridges, vaginal adenosis, cervical
D. (T) erosions, and clear-cell vaginal carcinoma than con-
E. (T) trol subjects. (Ref. 57)

245. A. (F) Transillumination of the scrotum helps identify cys-
B. (F) tic structures such as a hydrocele and a spermato-
C. (T) cele. A spermatocele is located above and separate
D. (F) from the testicle; a hydrocele surrounds the testicle.
E. (T) Thus, palpation usually allows the examiner to distinguish these cystic structures. (Ref. 114, p. 111)

The Head and Neck

246. (E) Hoarseness persisting for more than 2 weeks should be evaluated with laryngoscopy to rule out a neoplasm. (Ref. 37, p. 536)

247. (D) According to a caphalad–caudad orientation, the correct listing of midline neck structures is as follows: hyoid cartilage, thyroid cartilage, cricoid cartilage, and isthmus of the thyroid. (Ref. 8, p. 66)

248. (D) The feature that is most helpful in distinguishing the thyroid gland from other neck masses is its upward movement on swallowing. (Ref. 28, p. 211)

249. (A) A tracheal tug is seen with an aortic aneurysm. The dilated aorta's pulse wave may be palpated when the patient's neck is extended and the examiner lifts the trachea upward. (Ref. 95, p. 92)

250. (A) Using bedside techniques, several causes of unilateral cervical masses can be suspected. For example, a cystic hygroma can be transilluminated, a laryngocele increases in size when the patient exhales with the nose and mouth occluded, and gentle palpation of a carotid body tumor may produce pupillary dilatation. (Ref. 58, p. 240)

251. (D) Because a thyroglossal duct cyst connects with the base of the tongue through the thyroglossal duct, protrusion of the tongue results in an upward tug of the cyst. (Ref. 23, p. 162)

252. (D) A thyroid bruit strongly suggests the diagnosis of Graves' disease. (Ref. 92, p. 625)

253. (D) The general appearance of the head may be virtually pathognomonic for Paget's disease; characteristic findings include enlargement of the head with frontal bossing, dilated temporal arteries, and bruits audible over the bone. (Ref. 17, p. 39)

254. (D) The normal parotid gland is not palpable. It may be chronically enlarged in a variety of conditions, e.g., cirrhosis, diabetes mellitus, Sjögren's syndrome, neoplasms. (Ref. 95, p. 90)

255. A. (F)
B. (T)
C. (F)
D. (F)
E. (F)

The normal adult thyroid gland weighs about 30 g and is fixed to the trachea and larynx. The right lobe is usually larger than the left. The normal dimensions of the lateral lobe of the thyroid are about 5 cm × 3 cm × 2 cm. (Ref. 28, p. 210)

256. A. (F) Clinical features that suggest a thyroid nodule is ma-
B. (T) lignant include a history of childhood head and neck
C. (T) irradiation, occurrence in a male under 40 years of
D. (T) age, a solitary nodule, adjacent lymphadenopathy,
E. (T) fixation of the gland to adjacent structures, and a
hard consistency. (Ref. 122, p. 801)

257. A. (T) The differential diagnosis of facial edema includes
B. (T) hypoproteinemia, hypothyroidism, allergic reac-
C. (T) tions, trichinosis, and tricuspid stenosis. (Ref. 92,
D. (T) p. 170)
E. (T)

The Heart and Vessels

258. (D) Formerly, the first heart sound was thought to be caused by the closure of the atrioventricular valves (mitral and tricuspid). Current evidence suggests that the sound follows atrioventricular valve closure and is due to vibrations involving the valves, supporting structures, and ventricles. (Ref. 117, p. 63)

259. (D) A pulsus alternans is a regular alternating of weak and strong myocardial contractions that is independent of respiration and indicative of left ventricular failure. (Ref. 120, p. 735)

260. (E) Deep vein thrombosis is often silent. Because the clinical diagnosis of deep vein thrombosis is unreliable, confirmatory tests should be performed. The venogram is the most specific test. (Ref. 92, p. 1496)

261. (C) With a short PR interval, the AV valves are wide open at the end of diastole and then shut briskly at the onset of systole; this contributes to a loud S_1. (Ref. 60, p. 165)

262. (D) The external and internal jugular veins may be used as manometers to estimate right atrial pressure. The measurement should be expressed as cm of vertical distention or undulation above the angle of Louis with the patient's trunk in a specified position of elevation. (Ref. 91, p. 104)

263. (B) A sinus arrhythmia, an increase in heart rate with inspiration, is a frequent finding in normal young individuals. (Ref. 28, p. 361)

264. (A) The diastolic murmur of tricuspid stenosis is increased during inspiration because of the associated increase in flow across the tricuspid valve. (Ref. 117, p. 163)

265. (A) An S_4 is a low-pitched sound. (Ref. 120, p. 700)

266. (B) An S_4 is absent in the presence of atrial fibrillation. (Ref. 31, p. 254)

267. (E) The physical findings with angina pectoris are often normal; however, transient ischemia may produce left ventricular and papillary muscle dysfunction. (Ref. 92, p. 1426)

268. (A) A patient with chest pain who clenches his fist over the sternum while describing the pain should be evaluated for coronary heart disease. (Ref. 60, p. 890)

269. (E) Right atrial contraction produces the jugular venous "a" wave. (Ref. 2, p. 14)

270. (B) The auscultatory features of the normally functioning prosthetic mitral (ball) valve include a prominent opening click during early diastole and a closing sound that obscures S_1. A systolic ejection murmur is audible; a diastolic murmur is abnormal. (Ref. 107)

271. (C) The postphlebitic syndrome is characterized by dependent edema, increased pigmentation of the legs, cutaneous atrophy, and chronic ulcers. (Ref. 92, p. 1497)

272. (B) In patients with an acute inferior myocardial infarction, hemodynamically significant right ventricular infarction may be excluded if the jugular venous pressure is normal and Kussmaul's sign is absent. (Ref. 30)

273. (D) The cervical venous hum is frequently heard in normal children and adults. It is also associated with high output cardiac states. (Ref. 120, p. 614)

274. (D) Because the dorsalis pedis pulse may be congenitally absent in about 10% of patients, failure to palpate this pulse may not be clinically significant. (Ref. 120, p. 745)

275. (A) Advanced arteriosclerotic peripheral vascular disease causes ischemic injury to the microvasculature of the lower extremities. Reactive capillary dilatation produces chronic rubor of the extremity. (Ref. 110, p. 1983)

276. (D) A chronically very slow heart rate is characteristic of a third-degree atrioventricular block and an idioventricular escape rhythm. This is usually symptomatic, and a permanent pacemaker may be indicated. (Ref. 124, p. 320)

277. (E) Distended, nonpulsatile neck veins together with edema and cyanosis of the head, neck, and arms characterize the superior vena caval syndrome. (Ref. 28, p. 450)

278. (B) Pericarditis characteristically produces a tripartite scratching sound that corresponds to ventricular systole, ventricular diastole, and atrial systole. All three components may not always be present at one time in the same patient. (Ref. 120, p. 717)

279. (B) The term "ejection" murmur refers to a murmur produced by the forward flow of blood through a semilunar valve. Phonocardiographic studies document that these murmurs usually start with the tricuspid component of S_1; aortic ejection murmurs usually terminate prior to A_2, while pulmonic ejection murmurs usually terminate prior to P_2. (Ref. 26, p. 262)

280. (C) A left parasternal lift suggests right ventricular enlargement. (Ref. 60, p. 155)

281. (A) Patients with the straight back syndrome may demonstrate features suggestive of organic heart failure, e.g., a systolic ejection murmur, a delayed tricuspid valve closure sound, and expiratory splitting of the second sound. (Ref. 43, p. 103)

282. (C) The murmur of mitral valve prolapse is characteristically late systolic in timing. It is often preceded by a midsystolic click. (Ref. 92, p. 1410)

283. **(C)** The sternal angle of Louis is a useful reference point because in various positions it remains about 5 cm above the mid-right atrium. (Ref. 63, p. 159)

284. **(D)** The internal jugular vein is a more reliable indicator of venous wave form and venous pressure than the external jugular vein. Valves in the external system may interfere with retrograde pressure transmission. (Ref. 120, p. 654)

285. **(D)** The bell of the stethoscope is particularly useful for auscultating low-pitched sounds. If the examiner presses too hard with the bell, it is converted into a functional diaphragm. (Ref. 83, p. 124)

286. **(E)** While the internal jugular vein and carotid artery are in close proximity, only the vein is affected by posture, respiration, and gentle compression. (Ref. 120, p. 656)

287. **(C)** Severe central chest pain that radiates to the back and is not aggravated by changes in position or respiration suggests a dissecting aneurysm of the ascending aorta. (Ref. 10, p. 161)

288. **(E)** Jugular venous "a" waves are not seen with atrial fibrillation. (Ref. 60, p. 149)

289. **(E)** Thromboangitis obliterans (Buerger's disease) is a rare disease that affects young, male cigarette smokers. It is characterized by migratory thrombophlebitis and claudication of the distal extremities. (Ref. 92, p. 1494)

290. **(D)** In the ambulatory patient, minimal dependent edema may be first detected by palpating firmly just posterior to the medial malleolus. (Ref. 16, p. 257)

291. **(A)** The major value of cardiac percussion is to help identify situs inversus. In this situation, cardiac dullness and gastric tympany are percussed on the right while liver dullness is percussed on the left. (Ref. 91, p. 134)

292. (E) The most common cause of asymmetrical radial pules is an aberrant radial artery. Other causes, such as the thoracic outlet syndrome, are usually accompanied by signs and symptoms. (Ref. 45, p. 46)

293. (E) The location of the apical impulse in relation to the mid-sternal or midclavicular line is not an accurate indicator of left ventricular enlargement. In the left lateral decubitus position, an apical impulse greater than 3 cm may indicate left ventricular enlargement. (Ref. 36)

294. (C) The hepatojugular reflux may be useful in determining whether the venous pressure is elevated. With right heart failure, compression over the right upper quadrant forces blood into the chest and neck veins. (Ref. 43, p. 48)

295. (C) A patient with aortic atherosclerosis may develop atheroembolism manifest by hypertension, azotemia, livedo reticularis, and digital cyanosis. (Ref. 14, p. 1567)

296. (C) Total occlusion of the superficial, communicating, and deep venous systems of the leg is associated with cyanosis, edema, and absent or diminished arterial pulses in the involved extremity; this is phlegmasia cerulea dolens. (Ref. 28, p. 440)

297. (A) Clinical features are useful in distinguishing the systolic murmur of aortic stenosis from that of mitral regurgitation. With the former the murmur is louder after a premature ventricular depolarization. With the latter S_1 is often masked by the murmur, and S_2 is usually normal or widely split. (Ref. 45, p. 90)

298. (A) A patient with evidence of pulmonary hypertension and a loud S_1 should be carefully evaluated for mitral stenosis. (Ref. 14, p. 1068)

299. (E) The most useful clinical feature to distinguish aortic insufficiency from pulmonic insufficiency is peripheral evidence of aortic insufficiency, e.g., bounding pulses, and a wide pulse pressure. (Ref. 53, p. 211)

300. (B) The diagnosis of angina pectoris is established by a carefully performed interview. (Ref. 61, p. 1105)

301. (D) When chest pain is consistently precipitated by exertion and relieved by rest, myocardial ischemia should be suspected. Radiation of the pain down the left arm and relief of the pain by nitroglycerin are not specific for myocardial ischemia. (Ref. 92, p. 25)

302. (D) Positional changes in apical diastolic and systolic murmurs suggest the diagnosis of an atrial myxoma. (Ref. 60, p. 1287)

303. (B) Paradoxical splitting of S_2 is characterized by audible splitting during expiration with P_2 preceding A_2. (Ref. 3, p. 17)

304. (A) The intensity of murmurs is graded on a scale of 1 through 6. A grade 3 murmur is prominent, but not loud. (Ref. 60, p. 195)

305. (D) Peripheral pulse palpation is the most important physical diagnostic tool for establishing the diagnosis of arteriosclerotic peripheral vascular disease. (Ref. 46, p. 72)

306. (A) Primary lymphedema is characterized by symmetrical swelling of the toes, feet, and legs that does not pit. Initially, the skin appears normal, but verrucous changes may appear later. (Ref. 38, p. 1393)

307. (E) The thrill of aortic stenosis is best appreciated in the second interspace (left and right) with the patient leaning forward in expiration. (Ref. 14, p. 1099)

308. (C) A pulsus paradoxus is sought by listening for respiratory effects on the sounds of Korotkoff; a pulsus paradoxus is present if the systolic blood pressure varies by more than 8 mm Hg between expiration and inspiration. (Ref. 120, p. 516)

309. (B) Acute, peripheral arterial occlusion does not produce edema; this is useful in distinguishing arterial from venous disease. (Ref. 92, p. 1492)

310. (B) Innocent systolic murmurs probably originate in both the aortic and pulmonic valves. (Ref. 111)

311. (D) More than 4% of adult Americans over the age of 45 years demonstrate carotid artery bruits, and one-third of these are symptomatic. (Ref. 101)

312. (E) A supraclavicular systolic murmur is thought to arise because of increased flow through brachiocephalic arteries. It decreases or disappears with hyperextension of the shoulders. (Ref. 91, p. 214)

313. (E) The sphygmomanometer bladder width should equal 40% of the midarm circumference. For the average adult, a bladder width of 12–14 cm is appropriate. (Ref. 65)

314. (B) Pericardial rubs are heard best at the lower left sternal border. In some patients the rub is heard only when the patient is in the prone position, resting on the knees and elbows. (Ref. 91, p. 230)

315. (D) Mitral valve prolapse may produce no symptoms or may be associated with a variety of symptoms, e.g., nonexertional chest pain, palpitations, dizziness, weakness. The characteristic physical finding of this syndrome is a midsystolic click. (Ref. 61, p. 1098)

316. (B) The most common cause for a single S_2 is an inaudible P_2, which is most commonly seen in older patients with an increased anterior–posterior chest diameter. (Ref. 91, p. 183)

317. (D) Early diastolic sounds include the opening snap, a pericardial knock, a "tumor plop," and the mitral prosthetic sound. The S_3 is a middiastolic sound. (Ref. 91, p. 174)

318. (B) Late systolic, holosystolic, early diastolic, and holodiastolic murmurs are generally considered pathological. (Ref. 120, p. 708)

319. (C) The murmur of a patent ductus arteriosus is continuous. It begins with S_1, peaks near S_2, and then tapers off during diastole. (Ref. 91, p. 226)

320. (E) The murmur of acute severe aortic insufficiency differs significantly from that of chronic severe aortic insufficiency. The former is often short in duration, soft in intensity, medium in pitch, and impure in tone. (Ref. 91, p. 217)

321. (E) The following conditions may be associated with lateral displacement of the apical impulse in the absence of organic heart disease: pectus excavatum, congenital absence of the pericardium, elevated left hemidiaphragm, and pregnancy. (Ref. 120, p. 671)

322. A. (T)
B. (T)
C. (T)
D. (T)
E. (F)

Routine cardiac auscultation should include examination of the patient when he is supine, sitting, or standing, in the left lateral decubitus position, and after exercise. (Ref. 124, p. 152)

323. A. (T)
B. (T)
C. (T)
D. (T)
E. (F)

When a double-beating peripheral pulse is noted, the timing of the impulses should be noted. The double systolic pulse is a pulsus bisferiens and is seen with combined aortic stenosis and aortic insufficiency. When one impulse occurs in systole and the other occurs in diastole, this is a dicrotic pulse; this is seen in febrile states, with nonobstructive idiopathic cardiomyopathy, in healthy young people, and with cardiac tamponade. (Ref. 2, p. 41)

324. A. (F)
B. (T)
C. (T)
D. (T)
E. (F)

In patients over 40 years old, a third heart sound (S_3 gallop) usually indicates organic heart disease. (Ref. 120, p. 698)

325. A. (F)
B. (T)
C. (T)
D. (F)
E. (T)

Manifestations of aortic insufficiency include visible capillary pulsations, Duroziez's murmur, and the Austin Flint diastolic murmur. Capillary pulsations are not specific for aortic insufficiency. (Ref. 43, p. 569)

326. A. (T)
B. (F)
C. (T)
D. (T)
E. (F)

In an adult the zone of narrowing with coarctation of the aorta is usually distal to the origin of the left subclavian artery; hence, the blood pressure in the arms is usually the same. (Ref. 124, p. 237)

327. A. (F) Palpable beat-to-beat variations in peripheral pulse
B. (T) strength are seen with pulsus alternans and certain
C. (T) arrhythmias, e.g., bigeminy, and atrial fibrillation.
D. (F) (Ref. 8, p. 182)
E. (T)

328. A. (T) Although pulsus paradoxus is linked with cardiac
B. (T) tamponade, it is more frequently caused by asthma
C. (T) and pulmonary emphysema. It has also been re-
D. (T) ported in shock. (Ref. 43, p. 981)
E. (T)

329. A. (F) Differentiation of an innocent from an organic mur-
B. (F) mur may be difficult. Innocent murmurs tend to be
C. (T) systolic in timing, short in duration, and of soft in-
D. (F) tensity. (Ref. 43, p. 103)
E. (T)

330. A. (F) The major Jones criteria for making the diagnosis
B. (T) of rheumatic fever are erythema marginatum, sub-
C. (T) cutaneous nodules, polyarthritis, carditis, and cho-
D. (T) rea. (Ref. 92, p. 1399)
E. (F)

331. A. (T) Raynaud's disease is a vasospastic arterial disorder
B. (F) unassociated with systemic illness, which rarely
C. (T) causes digital ulceration. The sequential changes
D. (F) produced on cold exposure are pallor, cyanosis, and
E. (F) erythema, respectively. (Ref. 124, p. 353)

332. A. (F) A thrill is a palpable, organic murmur best timed by
B. (F) correlating it with the apical impulse. It is never a
C. (T) normal finding and only accompanies murmurs of
D. (F) moderate intensity or greater. (Ref. 28, p. 344)
E. (F)

333. A. (T) A faint diastolic rumble of mitral stenosis may only
B. (T) be heard at the apex in the left lateral position, as
C. (F) the patient moves into the left lateral position, or
D. (F) after exercise. (Ref. 43, p. 582)
E. (T)

334. A. (T) During a sustained Valsalva maneuver, the following
B. (F) events occur: the cardiac output falls, the systemic
C. (T) arterial blood pressure falls, the heart rate increases,
D. (F) the pulse pressure narrows, and the murmurs of idi-
E. (T) opathic hypertrophic subaortic stenosis and mitral
valve prolapse may increase. (Ref. 24)

335. A. (T) With complete heart block, ventricular tachycardia,
B. (F) and atrial fibrillation, the mitral and tricuspid valves
C. (F) are in varying positions at the time of their closure
D. (T) by ventricular contraction; this accounts for the vary-
E. (T) ing intensity of S_1. (Ref. 8, p. 193)

336. A. (F) The opening snap is a brief, high-pitched sound pro-
B. (F) duced by opening of the atrioventricular valves. It
C. (T) is most commonly associated with mitral stenosis,
D. (T) but it may also be heard with tricuspid stenosis and
E. (T) atrial tumors. (Ref. 95, p. 291)

337. A. (T) A systolic ejection click is an abnormal sound, but
B. (T) it does not necessarily indicate organic heart disease.
C. (F) It is usually due to abrupt opening of the semilunar
D. (F) valves or sudden distention of the great vessels.
E. (T) (Ref. 120, p. 706)

338. A. (T) Many disorders present as chest pain, e.g., an anx-
B. (T) iety reaction, costochondritis, osteoarthritis, mitral
C. (T) valve prolapse, and pericarditis; a meticulous phys-
D. (T) ical examination may reveal signs that point to a
E. (T) specific diagnosis. (Ref. 92, p. 25)

339. A. (T) Audible expiratory splitting of S_2 in the standing or
B. (T) sitting position suggests organic heart disease. Phys-
C. (F) iological splitting of S_2 is due both to an earlier A_2
D. (F) and a delayed P_2. (Ref. 102)
E. (F)

340. A. (F) The systolic ejection murmur of aortic stenosis is
B. (T) usually heard best at the second right intercostal

C. (T) space. It often radiates into the neck and may be
D. (F) heard best at the apex. (Ref. 43, p. 543)
E. (F)

341. A. (F) Pulsus parvus is a weak pulse associated with a narrow pulse pressure. It may be seen with cardiac tamponade, acute left ventricular failure, aortic stenosis, and mitral stenosis. (Ref. 95, p. 261)
B. (T)
C. (T)
D. (T)
E. (T)

342. A. (T) The apical impulse may not be palpable in 50% of older adults. In acutely ill patients with an absent apical impulse, pericardial tamponade should be considered. (Ref. 120, p. 671)
B. (F)
C. (T)
D. (F)
E. (T)

343. A. (F) Kussmaul's sign is an inspiratory distention of the neck veins that may be positive with constrictive pericarditis, severe right ventricular failure, and a restrictive cardiomyopathy. (Ref. 60, p. 148)
B. (F)
C. (F)
D. (T)
E. (T)

344. A. (T) A patient with hepatomegaly, distended neck veins, and ascites that is more prominent than dependent edema should be evaluated for chronic constrictive pericarditis. (Ref. 92, p. 1463)
B. (F)
C. (F)
D. (T)
E. (T)

345. A. (F) Allen's compression test is useful for demonstrating occlusive disease of the radial and ulnar arteries and the palmar arterial arch. (Ref. 60, p. 1340)
B. (F)
C. (T)
D. (T)
E. (T)

346. A. (T) An S_1 should be identified by correlating it with the upstroke of the carotid artery or the apical impulse. (Ref. 120, p. 681)
B. (F)
C. (T)
D. (F)
E. (F)

The Lymphatics

347. (A) A recent study developed a model to guide clinicians in deciding when to perform a biopsy on a peripheral lymph node in young patients. The clinical variables that were of greatest discriminant value were a lymph node greater than 2 cm in diameter; ear, nose, and throat symptoms; an abnormal chest x-ray. (Ref. 105)

348. (D) Focal sternal tenderness is a common finding with leukemia and has been reported with severe hemolytic anemia. The patient is usually unaware of its presence. (Ref. 123, p. 1511)

349. (C) The most common presenting manifestation of Hodgkin's disease is cervical and/or supraclavicular lymphadenopathy. (Ref. 123, p. 1654)

350. (B) The most common presenting sign with chronic myelocytic leukemia is splenomegaly. (Ref. 123, p. 1566)

351. (A) There are more than 500 lymph nodes in the body, and most of these are not accessible for physical examination. (Ref. 120, p. 623)

352. (A) Lymph nodes that measure more than 1.0 cm in diameter should be considered potentially abnormal. Lymph nodes measuring more than 3.0 cm in diameter should be checked for a neoplasm. (Ref. 46, p. 332)

353. (D) Lymph nodes measuring less than 1 cm in diameter may be normally palpated in the neck, axillary, and inguinal areas. (Ref. 46, p. 332)

354. A. (T)
B. (T)
C. (F)
D. (T)
E. (F)

Inguinal adenopathy is usually due to minor trauma or infection. Useful clinical information is not often obtained from a biopsy specimen at this site. (Ref. 46, p. 332)

355. **A. (T)** Carcinomatous lymph nodes tend to be very hard, bound to one another and to surrounding tissues, and nontender on palpation. (Ref. 123, p. 1280)
B. (F)
C. (F)
D. (F)
E. (T)

The Musculoskeletal System

356. **(C)** Myoedema is a transient, circumscribed elevation produced by striking a muscle. It is seen with hypothyroidism, debilitated states, and, occasionally, in normal people. (Ref. 75, p. 125)

357. **(D)** Relapsing polychondritis is an unusual connective tissue disease with a propensity for auricular and nasal cartilage involvement. (Ref. 76)

358. **(C)** A plantar neuroma is due to thickening of the third plantar common digital nerve in the web space. The patient experiences episodes of sharp pain and tenderness at this site. (Ref. 13, p. 418)

359. **(C)** Tennis elbow is due to chronic irritation of the wrist extensors' common origin at the lateral epicondyle of the humerus. (Ref. 59, p. 57)

360. **(E)** Very short fourth and fifth metacarpal and metatarsal bones are characteristic skeletal anomalies associated with pseudohypoparathyrodism and pseudopseudohypoparathyroidism. Patients with these disorders are hypocalcemic. (Ref. 92, p. 1942)

361. **(A)** In the presence of DeQuervain's disease (a stenosing tenosynovitis of the wrist) Finkelstein's test is positive. To perform the test, the patient makes a fist over the flexed thumb and the examiner deviates the hand in an ulnar direction. When this maneuver elicits pain at the styloid process, the test is positive. (Ref. 59, p. 77)

362. **(A)** A ganglion is a mucinous degeneration of the tendon sheath or joint capsule, which is usually translucent, fluctuant, round, and nontender. (Ref. 8, p. 358)

363. (B) Shoulder pain that is exacerbated by flexing and supinating the forearm against resistance suggests the diagnosis of bicipital tendinitis. (Ref. 63, p. 294)

364. (C) Ankylosing spondylitis should be suspected in a young man with pain and decreased mobility of the lumbar spine. Supportive findings include chest expansion of less than 2.5 cm and sacroiliac pain on joint compression. (Ref. 18)

365. (A) A patient whose knees are unusually close together and whose ankles are abnormally far apart has a genu valgus deformity. Valgus refers to the situation in which the apex of a deformity points toward the midline of the extremity; thus, with genu valgus, the knee deformity points toward the midline of the extremity. (Ref. 4, p. 15)

366. (D) Long, slender fingers (arachnodactyly) are seen in several conditions including: Marfan's syndrome, eunuchism, Ehlers–Danlos syndrome, and normal individuals with an asthenic habitus. (Ref. 64, p. 44)

367. (C) The metacarpophalangeal joint is rarely involved with osteoarthritis; its involvement is characteristic of rheumatoid arthritis. (Ref. 92, p. 2000)

368. (C) Chronic supraspinatus tendinitis is characterized by painful arm abduction between 60 degrees and 120 degrees. Point tenderness is also present between the greater and lesser humeral tuberosities. (Ref. 28, p. 709)

369. (A) Ischiogluteal bursitis presents with severe buttock pain. The diagnosis is established by demonstrating point tenderness at the ischial tuberosity. The straight leg raising test and Patrick's test may also be positive. (Ref. 28, p. 734)

370. (D) The anterior tibial compartment syndrome may develop a few hours after excessive exercise. It is characterized by anterior tibial pain, erythematous swelling, and loss of dorsiflexion of the great toe. (Ref. 23, p. 523)

371. (B) A goniometer, a modified protractor, should be used to accurately measure joint range of motion. (Ref. 11, p. 407)

372. (C) Painful, fusiform swelling of the proximal interphalangeal joints is characteristic of rheumatoid arthritis. (Ref. 31, p. 460)

373. (C) In the presence of a knee effusion, ballottement of the patella produces a clicking sensation as the patella strikes the femur. (Ref. 17, p. 208)

374. (A) Suprapubic pain seen with a positive obturator test identifies intrapelvic inflammation. The test is performed by flexing the thigh to 90 degrees, immobilizing the ankle with one hand, and rotating the knee medially and laterally with the other hand. (Ref. 28, p. 550)

375. (C) Measurement of the length of the leg should be made in the supine position from the anterior superior iliac spine to the medial malleolus. (Ref. 31, p. 462)

376. (B) With an extracapsular femoral fracture, the involved limb is characteristically shortened and externally rotated to 90 degrees. (Ref. 28, p. 743)

377. (D) Adson's test identifies compression of the brachial plexus and subclavian artery by the scalenus muscles. It is performed by palpating the radial pulse as the patient raises and turns his or her chin to one side and holds his or her breath in inspiration. (Ref. 28, p. 429)

378. (E) The Osgood–Schlatter syndrome is an apophysitis of the tibial tuberosity that presents with tenderness and swelling at this site. (Ref. 13, p. 392)

379. (B) Chondromalacia of the patella presents as attacks of knee pain. Examination reveals tenderness as the patella is pressed against the condyles and patellar crepitus with joint motion. (Ref. 28, p. 752)

380. (A) The history of finger trauma together with the inability to voluntarily extend the distal phalanx establishes the diagnosis of a mallet finger. This is due to rupture of the extensor tendon to the distal phalanx. (Ref. 28, p. 674)

381. (D) A line drawn between the iliac crests passes between the dorsal spines of lumbar vertebrae L-3 and L-4. A lumbar puncture may be safely performed below this level. (Ref. 83, p. 112)

382. (D) Scoliosis is a lateral curvature of the spine with an associated rotation of the vertebral bodies upon one another. (Ref. 13, p. 313)

383. (B) Recurrent hemarthroses are characteristic of hereditary disorders of coagulation, e.g., hemophilia and Christmas disease. (Ref. 92, p. 1901)

384. (E) Dupuytren's contracture is a disorder of unknown cause that presents with nodularity and contraction of the palmar fascia; this leads to flexion contractures of the proximal interphalangeal joints. (Ref. 88)

385. **A.** (T)
B. (T)
C. (T)
D. (T)
E. (T)

Hypertrophic osteoarthropathy may be idiopathic or associated with specific diseases, e.g., pulmonary tumors. Its clinical features may include bone deposition, periostitis, clubbing, synovitis, and arthritis. (Ref. 92, p. 2006)

386. **A.** (F)
B. (F)
C. (F)
D. (T)
E. (T)

Although the cause of a popliteal cyst (Baker's) is unknown, it is frequently associated with rheumatoid and degenerative arthritis. (Ref. 94, p. 226)

387. **A.** (T)
B. (F)
C. (T)
D. (F)
E. (T)

Myotonia dystrophica is a rare inherited disorder that may be first noted because the patient is unable to release his or her grasp after shaking hands. Cardiomegaly, cataracts, and testicular atrophy are also seen. (Ref. 92, p. 2189)

388. A. (F)
B. (F)
C. (F)
D. (F)
E. (F)

An anterior cruciate ligament tear gives a positive anterior drawer sign. A medial collateral ligament injury allows increased knee mobility on abducting the lower leg. (Ref. 59, p. 185)

389. A. (F)
B. (T)
C. (T)
D. (F)
E. (T)

Subcutaneous nodules located over bony prominences are seen with rheumatoid arthritis, rheumatic fever, and systemic lupus erythematosus. (Ref. 28, p. 658)

390. A. (T)
B. (T)
C. (T)
D. (T)
E. (F)

The temporomandibular joint may be successfully palpated either through the external auditory canal or anterior to the tragus. Simultaneous palpation may document asymmetrical movement, clicking, crepitation, and dislocation. (Ref. 59, p. 128)

391. A. (F)
B. (T)
C. (F)
D. (F)
E. (T)

"Fibrositis" refers to a poorly understood symptom complex of diffuse myalgias, stiffness, and fatigue. Tender "trigger points" and scapular skinfold tenderness are seen on physical examination. (Ref. 77, p. 1083)

392. A. (T)
B. (F)
C. (F)
D. (F)
E. (F)

A myopathy is characterized by proximal muscle weakness, absence of a sensory loss or fasciculations, and a late decrease in the deep tendon reflexes. (Ref. 6, p. 218)

393. A. (T)
B. (F)
C. (F)
D. (T)
E. (T)

The normal range of motion of the following joints is elbow flexion to 150 degrees, knee flexion to 135 degrees, ankle dorsiflexion to 20 degrees, shoulder abduction to 90 degrees, and hip extension to 30 degrees. (Ref. 11, p. 411)

394. A. (T)
B. (F)
C. (T)
D. (F)
E. (T)

Features of carpal spasm include wrist flexion, thumb flexion on the palm of the hand, finger adduction, metacarpophalangeal flexion, and interphalangeal joint extension. (Ref. 28, p. 665)

395. A. (F) Four objective signs of low back pain include loss
B. (T) of lumbar lordosis, a list of the lumbar spine, spasm
C. (T) of the erector spinae, and decreased range of lumbar
D. (T) spine motion. (Ref. 95, p. 461)
E. (T)

The Nervous System

396. (E) The abbreviated neurologic examination is appropriate for patients without symptoms of neurologic dysfunction. It can be completed in 2–3 minutes and should include the following items: examination of pupils, ocular movements, and the ocular fundus; examination of tendon and plantar reflexes; examination of facial movement and speech; examination of the strength of arm and leg muscles; examination of pain and vibratory sensation in the hands and feet. (Ref. 92, p. 67)

397. (A) Ataxic breathing is grossly irregular and suggests dysfunction at the level of the medulla. (Ref. 120, p. 846)

398. (B) Amaurosis fugax is an episode of monocular blindness that usually lasts less than 10 minutes and that suggests the diagnosis of a transient ischemic attack. (Ref. 81)

399. (E) The carpal tunnel syndrome is due to entrapment of the median nerve. Early clinical recognition is important because of the excellent surgical results. (Ref. 92, p. 2010)

400. (C) Decreased or absent deep tendon reflexes may be seen in disorders of the muscle, the myoneural junction, the anterior horn cell, and the peripheral nerve. Pyramidal tract disease produces hyperactive deep tendon reflexes. (Ref. 29, p. 442)

401. (E) Meralgia paresthetica is an entrapment neuropathy involving the lateral femoral cutaneous nerve in the fascia lata. It presents with lateral thigh pain and paresthesias. (Ref. 92, p. 2167)

402. (D) Ptosis usually results from a lesion of the third cranial nerve, the cervical sympathetic fibers, or the neuromuscular junction. (Ref. 31, p. 172)

403. (A) The characteristic gait of Parkinson's disease is festinating, i.e., an involuntary tendency to walk progressively faster. (Ref. 120, p. 966)

404. (D) The Romberg test primarily evaluates function of the posterior columns. (Ref. 29, p. 395)

405. (A) The abdominal and cremasteric reflexes are characteristically absent caudal to a pyramidal tract lesion. (Ref. 28, p. 810)

406. (D) Akathisia, i.e., motor restlessness, has been described in Parkinson's disease, postencephalitic states, and in patients receiving phenothiazines. (Ref. 29, p. 416)

407. (E) Asterixis is a "flapping" wrist movement that may be seen with several metabolic disorders including hepatic encephalopathy, uremia, carbon dioxide retention, and hypokalemia. (Ref. 120, p. 978)

408. (A) Clinical signs are predictive of future functional status in patients presenting with ischemic–hypoxic coma. Patients, who on initial examination demonstrate absent pupillary light reflexes, are highly unlikely to achieve independent, functional recovery. (Ref. 71)

409. (C) A retinal arteriolar cholesterol embolus appears as a small white or yellow plaque at an arteriolar bifurcation and is virtually diagnostic of carotid artery atherosclerosis. (Ref. 120, p. 613)

410. (B) The first sign of uncal herniation is usually ipsilateral pupillary dilatation. (Ref. 29, p. 161)

411. (C) Irritation of the first sacral root by a herniated disk characteristically produces a decreased Achilles tendon reflex, weakness of the plantar flexors, hypesthesia of the fifth toe, and posterior thigh pain. (Ref. 92, p. 39)

412. (A) Patients with the acute onset of low back pain should be examined for saddle anesthesia, cross-over leg pain, and absent anal sphincter tone; these findings strongly suggest the diagnosis of acute central disk herniation. (Ref. 51)

413. (B) Many tremors are exacerbated by purposeful movements such as the cerebellar and senile tremors. Occasionally, such tremors are referred to as "intention" tremors. (Ref. 75, p. 111)

414. (D) Spontaneous visible muscular twitches, fasciculations, suggest lower motor neuron disease. When they occur without other evidence of neurologic dysfunction, they may be benign. (Ref. 75, p. 123)

415. (B) A cervical sympathetic lesion may result in ptosis, miosis, enophthalmos, anhidrosis, and flushing on the involved side; this is Horner's syndrome. (Ref. 29, p. 129)

416. (D) Apraxia is a nonparalytic disorder in which the patient is unable to perform purposeful movements. (Ref. 92, p. 89)

417. (D) Anosognosia suggests a lesion involving the minor parietal lobe. (Ref. 92, p. 154)

418. (D) The posterior tibial nerve passes under the medial malleolus in the tarsal tunnel. It supplies sensory innervation to the heel, the sole, and the toes. Compression of this nerve in the tarsal tunnel, which is usually secondary to trauma, may produce paresthesias, nerve tenderness on palpation, and delayed nerve conduction time. Weakness and atrophy of the flexors of the toes may develop later. (Ref. 94, p. 265)

419. (D) A positive pronator sign suggests corticospinal tract disease. The patient is asked to shut his eyes and extend his arms in a supinated position; a positive pronator sign is present when there is downward drift and pronation of one arm. (Ref. 95, p. 412)

420. (A) Cherry-red skin color in a comatose patient suggests the diagnosis of carbon monoxide poisoning. (Ref. 92, p. 1265)

421. (B) Inability to perform rapid alternating movement is called dysdiadochokinesia. The presence of this abnormality suggests cerebellar dysfunction. (Ref. 114, p. 332)

422. (B) With a basilar skull fracture, bleeding from the posterior auricular artery may occur over the mastoid process (Battle's sign). (Ref. 29, p. 693)

423. (D) The ability to draw simple objects is a useful tool to evaluate constructional skills. Deficits in this ability strongly suggest a nondominant parietal lobe lesion. (Ref. 113, p. 102)

424. (B) The wakeful state is dependent upon interaction between the cerebral hemispheres and the reticular activating system. The reticular activating system extends from the medulla to the thalmus, but its caudal components do not appear essential for the wakeful state. (Ref. 93, p. 11)

425. (E) The diagnosis of benign positional vertigo can be confirmed at the bedside by a maneuver that reproduces the symptoms and produces transient nystagmus. In this maneuver the patient suddenly assumes the supine position with his head turned to one side. Vertigo and nystagmus appear for about 15 seconds. Going from the recumbent to the erect position reverses the direction of the nystagmus and vertigo. (Ref. 92, p. 85)

426. (A) Nasal speech suggests the diagnosis of soft palatal paralysis. The vagus nerve supplies motor innervation to the soft palate. (Ref. 29, p. 233)

427. (A) Nystagmoid movements are irregular, jerking, eye movements elicited on extreme lateral gaze in many normal individuals. (Ref. 92, p. 110)

428. (A) Myoclonus refers to a group of involuntary movement disorders that are rapid, brief, and purposeless. Some of the movements may be localized to an extremity, whereas others may be generalized. Myoclonus may be precipitated by external stimuli such as a loud sound. (Ref. 92, p. 97)

429. (D) Aphasia is a broad term that refers to the loss of communicative ability through speech or written language. The defect may be global or may refer to more selective problems in comprehension or production of speech and language. (Ref. 92, p. 145)

430. (C) Although a positive Kernig's sign is not specific for meningitis, it is a useful indicator of meningeal irritation. It is elicited by passively extending one leg on a flexed thigh. A positive sign is indicated by pain in the hamstring muscles and resistance to extension. (Ref. 29, p. 483)

431. (A) A broad-based, ataxic gait and inability to perform the heel-to-knee-to-toe test are seen with cerebellar degeneration. (Ref. 120, p. 969)

432. (A) Vertical nystagmus suggests a lesion in the brainstem. (Ref. 17, p. 219)

433. (A) Approximately 95% of the population is right-handed and demonstrates left cerebral dominance. Noting right or left handedness is important when evaluating disorders of language, especially aphasia. (Ref. 92, p. 145)

434. (D) Lesions of the posterior columns may produce an ataxic gait that is most apparent when visual clues are eliminated, i.e., when the patient walks with his eyes closed. (Ref. 29, p. 422)

435. (B) A lesion that completely destroys the right optic tract produces a left homonymous hemianopsia. (Ref. 92, p. 107)

436. (B) Involuntary, slow, snakelike movements of the extremities are characteristic of athetosis. (Ref. 75, p. 112)

437. (A) Orthostatic hypotension is the cardinal sign of idiopathic autonomic insufficiency; this is defined as a 30/20 mm Hg drop in the blood pressure upon assuming the erect position. Other associated signs may be present, such as absence of sinus arrhythmia and anhidrosis. (Ref. 124, p. 2028)

438. (E) Evaluation of station is accomplished with the patient standing with the feet close together. (Ref. 25, p. 420)

439. (E) Chvostek's sign indicates tetany and is due to hypocalcemia and hypomagnesemia. It is elicited by percussing the facial nerve just anterior to the external auditory meatus and observing for facial muscle contraction. (Ref. 92, p. 1942)

440. (B) Apneustic breathing is characterized by pauses at full inspiration. Most commonly, 2–3 second, end-inspiratory pauses occur with brief end-expiratory pauses. This type of breathing suggests damage to the respiratory centers in the pons. (Ref. 93, p. 38)

441. (C) Subtle neurological signs may occur in otherwise healthy, older individuals, including dorsal interosseous atrophy, slight intention tremor, loss of vibratory perception in the distal lower extremities, and some loss of associated movements. (Ref. 31, p. 94)

442. (D) The characteristic feature of vertigo is a rotational sensation. (Ref. 92, p. 82)

443. (B) A conservative approach to managing patients with an asymptomatic carotid bruit is justified. Patients should be followed up with noninvasive monitoring until the vessel diameter is reduced by 80%, or until patients become symptomatic; at that time, surgical treatment is indicated. (Ref. 98)

444. (C) The findings associated with a lower motor neuron lesion include muscular atrophy, weakness, fasciculations, hyporeflexia, and an absent or flexor plantar reflex. (Ref. 95, p. 399)

445. (B) True clonus indicates pyramidal tract disease. It is elicited in the ankle by dorsiflexing the foot; this produces sustained, rhythmic, alternating flexion and extension of the foot. (Ref. 29, p. 451)

446. (D) A tongue tremor may be seen with several conditions including anxiety, thyrotoxicosis, delirium tremens, and Parkinson's disease. (Ref. 28, p. 159)

447. (A) The spastic paraplegic patient moves each leg slowly and stiffly with a scissorlike movement due to strong hip adduction. The movements are awkward and the feet scuff along the floor. This type of gait may be seen with several disorders, including spinal tumors, spinal cord compression, and multiple sclerosis. (Ref. 92, p. 102)

448. (B) Every patient with neck pain and fever should be assessed for possible meningitis by testing for meningeal signs, e.g., Kernig's sign. (Ref. 46, p. 566)

449. (E) Lesions of selected peripheral nerves are correctly matched with their corresponding deficits as follows: long thoracic nerve—winging of the scapula; ulner nerve—claw hand; radial nerve—wrist drop; tibial nerve—the tarsal tunnel syndrome. (Ref. 29, p. 551)

450. A. (F)
B. (T)
C. (T)
D. (T)
E. (F)

Testing for two-point discrimination, graphesthesia, and stereognosis evaluates cortical sensory function. (Ref. 92, p. 115)

451. A. (T)
B. (F)
C. (T)
D. (T)
E. (F)

Decorticate posturing in a comatose patient suggests higher cortical dysfunction. Adduction and flexion of the arms and extension of the legs characterize this posture. (Ref. 120, p. 848)

452. A. (T)
B. (T)
C. (T)
D. (T)
E. (T)

Syringomyelia is a cavitary degeneration of the spinal cord that produces a characteristic dissociation of pain and touch perception. (Ref. 92, p. 2147)

453. A. (T)
B. (F)
C. (F)
D. (F)
E. (T)

Intact ciliospinal, oculocephalic, and oculovestibular reflexes are noted in the comatose patient with normal brainstem function. In the comatose patient, the normal caloric response is tonic ocular deviation toward the side of cold stimulation. (Ref. 92, p. 126)

454. A. (F)
B. (T)
C. (T)
D. (T)
E. (T)

Snout and suck reflexes are normal in infants. In adults they are associated with bilateral frontal lobe disease, corticobulbar disease, and coma. (Ref. 120, p. 981)

455. A. (T) Selected tendon reflexes are innervated as follows:
B. (T) C5-6, brachioradialis—C5-6, triceps—C6-8, patel-
C. (F) lar—L2-4, and Achilles—L5-S2. (Ref. 75, p. 172)
D. (F)
E. (F)

456. A. (F) The corneal reflex measures both fifth and seventh
B. (T) cranial nerve function and is affected by either pe-
C. (T) ripheral or central lesions. Normally, both eyes blink
D. (T) when the cornea of either eye is stimulated. (Ref.
E. (F) 63, p. 345)

457. A. (F) Persistent deviation of gait to one side suggests uni-
B. (T) lateral cerebellar or vestibular disease. (Ref. 29,
C. (F) p. 422)
D. (F)
E. (T)

458. A. (T) Opticokinetic nystagmus is a physiologic nystagmus
B. (F) that occurs while observing a moving object. Its ab-
C. (F) sence suggests a parietal lobe lesion. Its presence
D. (T) establishes that a patient is not blind. (Ref. 29,
E. (F) p. 149)

459. A. (T) Doll's eye movements, conjugate deviation of the
B. (T) eyes away from the direction in which the head is
C. (T) passively turned, are a useful indicator of an intact
D. (F) brainstem in the comatose adults. (Ref. 93, p. 54)
E. (T)

460. A. (F) The Babinski sign in adults is an abnormal superficial
B. (F) reflex suggesting the presence of pyramidal tract dis-
C. (T) ease. It should be elicited with the knee extended.
D. (F) It consists of extension of the great toe, and it is
E. (F) often accompanied by fanning of the other toes.
(Ref. 29, p. 456)

461. A. (F) Lhermitte's sign, the occurrence of electriclike sen-
B. (T) sations passing down the body with neck flexion,
C. (F) occurs with multiple sclerosis, cervical spine disk dis-

D. (T) ease, and cervical spine neoplasms. (Ref. 29, p. 582)
E. (T)

462. A. (T) A completely positive Hoffman sign includes flexion and adduction of the thumb and flexion of the index finger. It is an indicator of hyperactive muscle stretch reflexes. (Ref. 29, p. 453)
B. (F)
C. (F)
D. (F)
E. (F)

463. A. (T) Correct sensory innervation includes the face—the fifth cranial nerve, the neck—C-3, the nipple—T-5, the great toe—L-5, the fifth toe—S-1. (Ref. 92, p. 8)
B. (F)
C. (T)
D. (F)
E. (F)

464. A. (T) The "flapping tremor" of hepatic encephalopathy disappears at rest and with hepatic coma. It is reduced by purposeful movement and exacerbated by sustained posture. (Ref. 103, p. 92)
B. (F)
C. (T)
D. (F)
E. (T)

465. A. (T) When a blind eye is stimulated, the consensual light reflex is absent on the normal side. When the normal eye is stimulated, the consensual light reflex is intact in the blind eye if the oculomotor nerve is normal. (Ref. 29, p. 133)
B. (T)
C. (F)
D. (T)
E. (T)

466. A. (F) Tests of abstract thinking include interpretation of proverbs, interpretation of analogies, and explanation of similarities between objects. (Ref. 113, p. 108)
B. (F)
C. (T)
D. (T)
E. (T)

The Skin

467. (A) Petechiae suggest a platelet or vascular disorder and are rarely seen in coagulopathies. (Ref. 123, p. 1045)

468. (E) The heliotrope rash is a violet discoloration of the upper eyelid, which is characteristic of dermatomyositis. (Ref. 97, p. 67)

469. (A) Atopic eczema is a common chronic dermatitis characterized by areas of dry, crusted, and excoriated lesions. A chronic itch–scratch cycle is characteristic. A prominent family history of asthma or hay fever is common. The lesions are most often found on the face and antecubital fossa. (Ref. 40, p. 14)

470. (A) Skin tags may be cutaneous markers for colonic polyps and may thus help identify patients at increased risk for developing colon cancer. (Ref. 69)

471. (A) Multiple spider angiomas are most commonly associated with diffuse liver disease, e.g., cirrhosis. They are also seen with pregnancy, thyrotoxicosis, and in the normal state. (Ref. 92, p. 264)

472. (B) Periungual telangiectasias are characteristic of lupus erythematosus, dermatomyositis, and scleroderma. They have also been reported in patients exposed to vinyl chloride. (Ref. 15, p. 534)

473. (A) Characteristically, a basal cell carcinoma presents as a nodule with a pearllike surface and superficial telangiectasia. Biopsy is necessary for diagnosis. (Ref. 112, p. 537)

474. (D) Axillary "freckles" are small *cafe au lait* spots measuring 1–4 mm and are diagnostic of neurofibromatosis. (Ref. 15, p. 789)

475. (C) Hidradenitis suppurativa is a disorder of apocrine glands that results in chronic inflammation and scarring. Early diagnosis markedly improves the therapeutic response. (Ref. 38, p. 480)

476. (E) Bullous lesions in sun-exposed areas characterize porphyria cutanea tarda. Recognition is important because treatment with phlebotomy is effective. (Ref. 124, p. 1157)

477. (C) Target lesions are diagnostic of erythema multiforme. They are characterized by an elevated, red circular border, an inner pale zone, and a central erythematous area. (Ref. 112, p. 212)

478. (E) Cyanosis from any of several causes is usually clinically apparent when more than 5 g% of unsaturated capillary hemoglobin is present. (Ref. 92, p. 162)

479. (B) Acanthosis nigricans presents as velvety, pigmented plaques in the axilla, groin, and umbilicus. When this condition develops in an adult in the absence of obesity and endocrinopathies, an underlying malignancy is usually present. (Ref. 92, p. 832)

480. (E) Focal hypopigmentation of scalp hair is seen with alopecia areata, piebaldism, vitiligo, and tuberous sclerosis. Albinism is associated with diffuse hypopigmentation of scalp hair. (Ref. 68, p. 487)

481. (E) When the pigmented macules of urticaria pigmentosa are rubbed, mast cells degranulate producing urticaria; this is Darier's sign and is virtually diagnostic for urticaria pigmentosa. (Ref. 38, p. 16)

482. (A) Erythema nodosum is associated with the use of oral contraceptives. The lesions are inflamed nodules, characteristically located on the anterior tibial surface. (Ref. 15, p. 476)

483. (E) Pyroderma gangrenosum is a spontaneously developing ulcerative disorder that may be associated with ulcerative colitis, Crohn's disease, collagen vascular diseases, and blood dyscrasias. It has characteristic features such as tender, raised margins that are undermined. (Ref. 68, p. 329)

484. (C) Scabies is due to a mite that burrows into the skin leaving threadlike lesions that are intensely pruritic. The webs of the fingers are often involved. (Ref. 124, p. 1838)

485. (D) Subcutaneous crepitus is the unique sensation imparted to the fingers upon palpating bubbles of air or gas in the subcutaneous tissue or muscle. It is found with subcutaneous emphysema and gas gangrene. (Ref. 28, p. 502)

486. (C) Perifollicular hyperkeratosis and petechiae are suggestive of scurvy; corkscrew-appearing hairs that become buried in the follicles are also seen with scurvy. (Ref. 123, p. 147)

487. (E) Trauma is probably the most common cause of onycholysis. (Ref. 38, p. 424)

488. (C) Both Osler's nodes and Janeway lesions are cutaneous manifestations of endocarditis. Osler's node is painful, whereas the Janeway lesion is nontender. (Ref. 38, p. 1401)

489. (B) Beau's lines are transverse nail grooves that may be useful in dating a severe illness. (Ref. 120, p. 543)

490. (D) Pinpoint nail crypts may be found in patients with psoriasis. This abnormality is seen more commonly in psoriatic patients with arthritis. (Ref. 17, p. 121)

491. (D) Unilateral clubbing and unidigital clubbing are seen with localized vascular lesions, e.g., an arteriovenous fistula. (Ref. 38, p. 430)

492. (A) Koilonychia, spoon nail, is seen most often with iron deficiency anemia. (Ref. 28, p. 686)

493. (A) Flattening of the angle between the proximal nail plate and the dorsal surface of the finger is the single best clinical finding establishing the diagnosis of clubbing. (Ref. 120, p. 730)

494. (E) The acute dermatitis–arthritis syndrome of gonococcemia is probably the most common cause of acute arthritis in young adults. (Ref. 92, p. 900)

495. (B) A dermatofibroma may be confused with a melanoma. Differentiation may be accomplished by applying lateral digital pressure; the dermatofibroma "dimples," whereas a melanoma protrudes above the skin. (Ref. 39)

496. (D) A glomus tumor is a benign growth of a normally occurring arteriovenous anastomosis of the finger. It is often located under the nail and is very tender on palpation. (Ref. 23, p. 477)

497. (B) Cherry angiomas are bright-red papules, measuring 2–3 mm in diameter, that do not blanch. They are common in older adults, and are not associated with systemic illness. (Ref. 123, p. 1075)

498. (D) Diffusely yellow nails are related to impaired lymphatic drainage, e.g., primary lymphedema. (Ref. 112, p. 403)

499. (D) Multiple, 2–5-mm, brown macules on the lips, buccal mucosa, and dorsum of the fingers suggest the diagnosis of the Peutz–Jeghers syndrome. The gastrointestinal polyps seen with this syndrome do not have a high rate of malignant degeneration. (Ref. 38, p. 608)

500. (E) A keratoacanthoma is a benign tumor that is thought to arise from hair follicles. Although it may be confused with a carcinoma, its rapid growth allows accurate clinical recognition. (Ref. 38, p. 383)

501. (B) Psoriasis is characterized by the Koebner reaction (development of scaling plaques at sites of trauma) and the Auspitz sign (production of punctate bleeding points by abrading the scaly plaque). (Ref. 38, p. 236)

502. (D) In general, when the palmar creases lose their pink color, the hemoglobin concentration is 7 g/dL or less. (Ref. 123, p. 534)

503. (B) Early recognition of the clinical forms of melanoma greatly enhances survival. Lentigo maligna melanoma begins as a large frecklelike lesion that enlarges over a period of years and develops multiple areas of increased and decreased pigmentation. (Ref. 38, p. 635)

504. (A) A plantar wart presents as a dark core that is very painful when compressed against adjacent bony structures. Accompanying tiny, dark, superficial spots are due to thrombosed verrucous vessels. (Ref. 23, p. 542)

505. (D) Impetigo is a pyoderma that is usually caused by streptococci. The initial lesions are vesicles, which subsequently form characteristic yellow, "stuck-on" crusts. (Ref. 38, p. 1428)

506. (B) Pityriasis rosea is an acute maculopapular exanthem that is usually preceded by a 2–5-cm erythematous, scaling lesion, the herald patch. (Ref. 40, p. 74)

507. (D) A hard, hyperkeratotic skin projection seen in elderly patients is a cutaneous horn. This is a premalignant lesion. (Ref. 112, p. 512)

508. (B) Carotenemia is manifest by a diffuse yellow appearance of the skin and normal appearing sclerae. It results from eating excessive carotene-containing foods and is harmless. (Ref. 92, p. 469)

509. (A) Subcutaneous lipomata may often be clinically recognized because of their lobulated texture on palpation. (Ref. 23, p. 23)

510. (C) Actinic keratoses are common premalignant skin lesions. (Ref. 92, p. 835)

511. (A) Patients with myxedema have dry, coarse hair. (Ref. 31, p. 130)

512. (A) Ossification of the skin or subcutaneous tissue is seen in a variety of conditions including skin tumors, hypoparathyroidism, and neurologic disorders. (Ref. 38, p. 1137)

513. (E) "Palpable" (papular) purpura is usually due to very serious problems, and the underlying cause should be vigorously sought. The differential diagnosis includes systemic vasculitis, endocarditis, consumption coagulopathy, and Rocky Mountain spotted fever. (Ref. 68, p. 347)

514. (A) Hyperpigmentation in scars and creases is characteristic of Addison's disease. (Ref. 46, p. 677)

515. (D) The sudden appearance of numerous seborrheic keratoses may be an indicator of internal malignancy, usually gastric carcinoma. This is the sign of Leser–Trelat. (Ref. 27)

516. (A) The papules seen with amyloidosis often demonstrate spontaneous hemorrhage, or hemorrhage after minimal trauma, i.e., "pinch purpura." (Ref. 38, p. 1064)

517. (B) Tendon xanthomas suggest the diagnosis of type II hyperlipoproteinemia; they characteristically involve the Achilles and patellar tendons, as well as tendons on the plantar surface of the feet and dorsum of the hands. (Ref. 92, p. 554)

518. A. (T)
B. (F)
C. (F)
D. (F)
E. (T)

The normal "flesh" skin color is determined by four pigments (melanin, oxyhemoglobin, reduced hemoglobin, and carotene) and by an optical effect, scattering. Scattering directs incident blue rays back to the surface of the skin where they combine with reflected red rays to produce the "flesh" color. (Ref. 10, p. 814)

519. A. (F)
B. (T)
C. (T)
D. (T)
E. (T)

Among skin disorders, melanoma is the leading cause of death. Early identification contributes to improved diagnosis. Variegated color, irregular margins, and an irregular surface are indications for biopsy. (Ref. 92, p. 836)

520. A. (T)
B. (F)
C. (F)
D. (T)
E. (T)

Identification of primary skin lesions precedes specific dermatologic diagnosis. A macule is a common primary lesion due to a change in skin color. It is circumscribed and not elevated. (Ref. 92, p. 249)

521. A. (T)
B. (T)
C. (T)
D. (T)
E. (T)

Subungual splinter hemorrhages are associated with several conditions including bacterial endocarditis, trauma, trichinosis, mitral stenosis, and the normal state. (Ref. 38, p. 1435)

522. A. (F)
B. (F)
C. (T)
D. (F)
E. (F)

Alopecia areata is a sudden, patchy loss of hair that may involve the scalp, beard, and eyebrows. Nail dystrophy may accompany this disorder. (Ref. 112, p. 234)

523. A. (T)
B. (T)
C. (T)

Telangiectasias are composed of dilated arterioles, capillaries, or venules. They are a characteristic feature of actinically damaged skin, necrobiosis lipoid-

D. (F) ica, acne rosacea, and radiation dermatitis. (Ref. 15,
E. (T) p. 532)

524. A. (T) Nail hypertrophy may be a congenital abnormality,
B. (T) but it is also associated with vascular insufficiency,
C. (T) fungal infections, trauma, and psoriasis. (Ref. 112,
D. (T) p. 407)
E. (T)

525. A. (T) Flushing is due to paroxysmal vasodilatation. This
B. (T) may be mediated by biologically active substances
C. (T) or by vasomotor nerves. The differential diagnosis
D. (T) includes carcinoid syndrome, systemic mastocytosis,
E. (T) medullary thyroid carcinoma, menopause, and emotional stimuli. (Ref. 92, p. 823)

526. A. (T) Generalized erythematous scaling (erythroderma
B. (T) syndrome) may be associated with a drug reaction,
C. (T) a lymphoma, leukemia, psoriasis, and atopic der-
D. (T) matitis. (Ref. 92, p. 258)
E. (T)

527. A. (T) Vitiligo is a heritable hypomelanosis of the skin,
B. (T) hair, and mucosa. Lesions often develop in areas of
C. (T) trauma. Patients are usually asymptomatic. (Ref. 38,
D. (T) p. 582)
E. (T)

528. A. (T) The dysplastic nevus syndrome is a heritable disor-
B. (T) der in which atypical nevi have an increased risk of
C. (T) malignant transformation. Clinical characteristics of
D. (T) these nevi include size larger than 6 mm, variegated
E. (T) color ranging from tan to brown on a red background, irregular borders and surface, and location in both sun-exposed and sun-protected areas. (Ref. 47)

529. A. (T) Arsenical toxicity is associated with an increased risk
B. (T) of developing Bowen's disease of the skin, a squa-
C. (F) mous cell carcinoma, a basal cell carcinoma, and
D. (T) internal malignancies. (Ref. 15, p. 71)
E. (T)

The Vital Signs

530. (E) According to the American Heart Association, the true intraarterial diastolic blood pressure in adults corresponds closely to that point in which the Korotkoff sounds become inaudible (fifth phase). (Ref. 65)

531. (E) In the presence of the auscultatory gap due to an absent second phase of Korotkoff, inaccurately low systolic, or high diastolic blood pressure measurements may be obtained. (Ref. 8, p. 183)

532. (A) Unless an obesity cuff is used, artifactually elevated blood pressure measurements may be obtained in obese patients. (Ref. 17, p. 47)

533. (B) The sounds of Korotkoff can be amplified through decreasing the venous pressure in the arm. (Ref. 63, p. 153)

534. (C) Normally, upon assuming the erect position, the systolic blood pressure may drop 10 mm Hg and the diastolic blood pressure may rise 5 mm Hg. (Ref. 63, p. 153)

535. (C) Elderly patients may demonstrate spurious hypertension due to sclerotic vessels. A sclerotic brachial artery, which is palpable when the blood pressure cuff is inflated above the systolic pressure, helps identify individuals with this problem. (Ref. 79)

536. (B) The cessation of sound is the fifth phase of Korotkoff; it corresponds closely to the diastolic blood pressure. (Ref. 44, p. 55)

537. (C) The pulse pressure is the difference between the systolic and diastolic blood pressure and is normally between 30 and 40 mm Hg; it is narrowed with constrictive pericarditis. (Ref. 28, p. 401)

538. (C) Periodic (Cheyne–Stokes) respiration is characterized by apneic episodes followed by cycles of breathing. The latter begin slowly, peak with tachypnea and hyperpnea, and taper off to the apneic cycle. (Ref. 95, p. 197)

539. **(C)** Sighing respirations suggest the diagnosis of an anxiety reaction. (Ref. 28, p. 280)

540. **(D)** The mercury sphygmomanometer is recommended over the aneroid sphygmomanometer. The former is more accurate, reliable, and durable; in the long run it is also less costly to maintain. (Ref. 87, p. 20)

541. **(E)** The normal adult resting respiratory rate should not exceed 18 cycles/min. (Ref. 28, p. 278)

542. **(A)** When electronic digital thermometers are employed, tachypnea may mask the presence of clinical fever. In this setting rectal temperature measurements are more reliable. (Ref. 115)

543. **A. (T)** **B. (T)** **C. (T)** **D. (T)** **E. (T)** A pulse deficit is defined as the difference between the apical and peripheral pulse rates; it occurs whenever ventricular contraction occurs before ventricular filling adequate to produce a peripheral pulse. (Ref. 95, p. 255)

544. **A. (F)** **B. (T)** **C. (F)** **D. (F)** **E. (F)** When using a 20-cm bag and with the patient lying on his or her abdomen, the systolic blood pressure in the thigh is usually 10–40 mm Hg greater than and the diastolic blood pressure is nearly the same as in the arm. (Ref. 65)

545. **A. (T)** **B. (T)** **C. (T)** **D. (T)** **E. (T)** A patient with profound hypothermia may appear to be dead because the following physical findings may be present: an unobtainable pulse, rigid joints, apparently absent pupillary reflexes and respiration, and unresponsiveness to all external stimuli. (Ref. 82, p. 430)

546. **A. (T)** **B. (T)** **C. (F)** **D. (F)** **E. (T)** An occasional patient with fever of unknown origin may have "factitious fever"; this is suggested when the pulse and respiratory rate remain normal during febrile episodes, there is no diaphoresis after lysis of fever, and there is disagreement between the temperature of a freshly voided urine specimen and the rectal temperature. (Ref. 120, p. 40)

547. A. (F) The radial pulse should always be palpated while
B. (T) pumping up the sphygmomanometer cuff. Its obli-
C. (F) teration corresponds closely with the first phase of
D. (T) Korotkoff and the systolic blood pressure. (Ref. 60,
E. (T) p. 139)

548. A. (F) When taking the blood pressure, phases I, IV, and
B. (F) V of Korotkoff should be recorded. A very low pres-
C. (T) sure for phase V suggests the presence of a high-
D. (T) output cardiac state. (Ref. 60, p. 139)
E. (F)

549. A. (T) A wide pulse pressure is found in several disorders,
B. (T) including aortic insufficiency, peripheral arteriove-
C. (T) nous fistula, patent ductus arteriosus, and beriberi
D. (T) heart disease. (Ref. 28, p. 401)
E. (F)

550. A. (F) In an adult, a significant blood pressure difference
B. (T) between the arms may be an important clue for the
C. (T) diagnosis of the subclavian steal syndrome, the tho-
D. (T) racic outlet syndrome, and arteriosclerotic disease
E. (F) of the subclavian artery. (Ref. 60, p. 141)

References

1. American Academy of Ophthalmology and Otolaryngology: *Ophthalmology Study Guide*, 3rd ed., 1978.

2. American Heart Association: *Examination of the Heart*. Part two: Inspection and Palpation of Venous and Arterial Pulses. Dallas, 1978.

3. American Heart Association: *Examination of the Heart*. Part four: Auscultation. Dallas, 1974.

4. American Orthopaedic Association: *Manual of Orthopaedic Surgery*, 5th ed., Chicago, 1979.

5. Barker, L. R., et al.: *Principles of Ambulatory Medicine*, Williams & Wilkins Company, Baltimore, 1982.

6. Barondess, J. A.: *Diagnostic Approaches to Presenting Syndromes*, Williams & Wilkins Company, Baltimore, 1971.

7. Basmajian, J. V.: *Surface Anatomy*, William & Wilkins Company, Baltimore, 1977.

8. Bates, B.: *A Guide to Physical Examination*, 3rd ed., J. B. Lippincott Company, Philadelphia, 1983.

9. Baum, G. L.: *Textbook of Pulmonary Diseases*, 3rd ed., Little, Brown & Company, Boston, 1983.

10. Blacklow, R. S.: *MacBryde's Signs and Symptoms*, J. P. Lippincott Company, Philadelphia, 1983.

11. Bouchier, I. A. D. and Morris, J. S.: *Clinical Skills*, W. B. Saunders Company, Philadelphia, 1976.

12. Branch, W. T., Jr.: *Office Practice of Medicine*, W. B. Saunders Company, Philadelphia, 1982.

13. Brashear, H. R., Jr., and Raney, R. B., Sr.: *Shands' Handbook of Orthopedic Surgery*, 9th ed., C. V. Mosby Company, St. Louis, 1978.

14. Braunwald, E.: *Heart Disease*, 2nd ed., W. B. Saunders Company, Philadelphia, 1984.

15. Braverman, I. M.: *Skin Signs of Systemic Disease*, 2nd ed., W. B. Saunders Company, Philadelphia, 1981.

16. Buckingham, W. B. et al.: *A Primer of Clinical Diagnosis*, 2nd ed., Harper & Row Publishers, Hagerstown, 1979.

17. Burnside, J. W.: *Physical Diagnosis*, 16th ed., Williams & Wilkins Company, Baltimore, 1981.

18. Calabro, J. J. and Maltz, B. A.: Ankylosing, Spondylitis. *N Engl J Med* 282:606–610, 1970.

19. Carlson, H. E.: Gynecomastia. *N Engl J Med* 303:795–799, 1980.

20. Castell, D. O. et al.: Estimation of liver size by percussion in normal individuals. *Ann Intern Med* 70:1183–1189, 1969.

21. Cattau, E. L., et al.: The accuracy of the physical examination in the diagnosis of suspected ascites. *JAMA* 247:1164–1166, 1982.

22. Chawla, H. B.: *Essential Ophthalmology*, Churchill Livingstone, Edinburgh, 1981.

23. Clain, A.: *Hamilton Bailey's Demonstrations of Physical Signs in Clinical Surgery*, 16th ed., Williams & Wilkins Company, Baltimore, 1980.

24. Cochran, P. T.: Bedside aids to auscultation of the heart. *JAMA* 239:54–55, 1978.

25. Cogan, D. G.: *Ophthalmic Manifestations of Systemic Vascular Disease*, W. B. Saunders Company, Philadelphia, 1974.

26. Constant, J.: *Bedside Cardiology*, 2nd ed., Little, Brown & Company, Boston, 1976.

27. Dantzig, P. I.: Sign of Leser–Trelat. *Arch Dermatol* 108:700–701, 1973.

28. DeGowin, E. L. and DeGowin, R. L.: *Bedside Diagnostic Examination*, 4th ed., Macmillan Publishing Company, New York, 1981.

29. DeJong, R. N.: *The Neurologic Examination*, 4th ed., Harper & Row Publisher, New York, 1979.

30. Dellitalia, L. J., et al.: Physical examination for exclusion of hemodynamically important right ventricular infarction. *Ann Intern Med* 99:608–611, 1983.

31. Delp, M. H. and Manning, R. T.: *Major's Physical Diagnosis*, 9th ed., W. B. Saunders Company, Philadelphia, 1981.

32. DeWeese, D. D. and Saunders, W. H.: *Textbook of Otolaryngology*, 6th ed., C. V. Mosby Company, St. Louis, 1982.

33. Druger, G.: *The Chest: Its Signs and Sounds*, Humetrics Corporation, Inglewood, 1973.

34. Dyken, P. R. and Miller, M. D.: *Facial Features of Neurologic Syndromes*, C. V. Mosby Company, St. Louis, 1980.

35. Earnest, D. L. and Fletcher, G. F.: Danger of rectal examination in patients with acute myocardial infarction—fact or fiction? *N Engl J Med* 281:238–241, 1969.

36. Eilen, S. D., et al.: Accuracy of precordial palpation for detecting increased left ventricular volume. *Ann Intern Med* 99:628–630, 1983.

37. English, G. M.: *A Textbook of Otolaryngology*, Harper & Row Publishers, Hagerstown, 1976.

38. Fitzpatrick, T. B. et al: *Dermatology in General Medicine*, 2nd ed., McGraw–Hill Book Company, New York, 1979.

39. Fitzpatrick, T. B. and Gilchrest, B. A.: Dimple sign to differentiate benign from malignant pigmented cutaneous lesions. *N Engl J Med* 296:1518–1519, 1977.

40. Fitzpatrick, T. B., et al.: *Color Atlas and Synopsis of Clinical Dermatology*, McGraw–Hill Book Company, New York, 1983.

41. Fleming, C. R., et al.: Pigmented corneal rings in non-Wilsonian liver disease. *Ann Intern Med* 86:285–288, 1977.

42. Forgacs, P.: *Lung Sounds*. Bailliere Tindall, London, 1978.

43. Fowler, N. O.: *Cardiac Diagnosis and Treatment*, 3rd ed., Harper & Row Publishers, Hagerstown, 1980.

44. Frank, M. J. and Alvarez–Mena, S. V.: *Cardiovascular Physical Diagnosis*, Year Book Medical Publishers, Chicago, 1973.

45. Friedman, H. H.: *Problem-Oriented Medical Diagnosis*, 3rd ed., Little, Brown & Company, Boston, 1983.

46. Goroll, A. H., et al: *Primary Care Medicine*, J. P. Lippincott Company, Philadelphia, 1981.

47. Green, M. H. et al.: Acquired precursors of cutaneous malignant melanoma. *N Engl J Med* 312:91–97, 1985.

48. Greenspan, J. S., et al.: Replication of Epstein-Barr virus within the epithelial cells of oral "hairy" leukoplakia, an AIDS-associated lesion. *N Engl J Med* 313:1564–1570, 1985.

49. Guarina, J. R.: Auscultatory percussion of the chest. *Lancet*, 1980; i:1332–1334.

50. Haagensen, C. D.: *Diseases of the Breast*, 2nd ed., W. B. Saunders Company, Philadelphia, 1974.

51. Hall, H.: Examination of the patient with low back pain. *Bull Rheum Dis* 33:1–8, 1983.

52. Hardison, J. E.: Venous hum of Cruveilhier–Baumgarten syndrome. *Arch Intern Med* 137:1623–1624, 1977.

53. Harvey, A., Mc., et al.: *The Principles and Practice of Medicine*, 21st ed., Appleton–Century–Crofts, New York, 1983.

54. Havener, W. H.: *Synopsis of Ophthalmology*, 5th ed., C. V. Mosby Company, St. Louis, 1979.

55. Haynes, B. E., et al.: The diagnosis of testicular torsion. *JAMA* 249:2522–2527, 1983.

56. Heinz, G. J. and Zavala, D. C.: Slipping rib syndrome. *JAMA* 237:794–795, 1977.

57. Herbst, A. L., et al.: Prenatal exposure to stilbestrol. *N Engl J Med* 292:334–339, 1975.

58. Hillman, R. S., et al.: *Clinical Skills: Interviewing, History Taking and Physical Diagnosis*, McGraw–Hill Book Company, New York, 1981.

59. Hoppenfeld, S.: *Physical Examination of the Spine and Extremities*, Appleton–Century–Crofts, New York, 1976.

60. Hurst, J. W.: *The Heart*, 6th ed., McGraw–Hill Book Company, New York, 1986.

61. Hurst, J. W.: *Medicine for the Practicing Physician*, Butterworths, Boston, 1983.

62. Johnson, D. H. and Brubar, R. F.: Glaucoma: An overview. *Mayo Clin Proc* 61:59–67, 1986.

63. Judge, R. D. and Zuidema, G. D.: *Methods of Clinical Examination: A Physiologic Approach*, 3rd ed., Little, Brown & Company, Boston, 1974.

64. Judge, R. D., et al.: *Clinical Diagnosis*, 4th ed., Little, Brown & Company, Boston, 1982.

65. Kirkendall, W. M., et al.: Recommendations for human blood pressure determination by sphygmomanometers. *Circulation* 62:1146A–1155A, 1980.

66. Klein, L. A.: Prostatic carcinoma. *N Engl J Med* 300:824–833, 1979.

67. Komaroff, A. L., et al.: The prediction of streptococcal pharyngitis in adults. *J Gen Intern Med* 1:1–7, 1986.

68. Lazarus, G. S. and Goldsmith, L. A.: *Diagnosis of Skin Disease*, F. A. Davis Company, Philadelphia, 1980.

69. Leavitt, J., et al.: Skin tags: A cutaneous marker for colonic polyps. *Ann Intern Med* 98:928–930, 1983.

70. Lehrer, S.: *Understanding Lung Sounds*, W. B. Saunders Company, Philadelphia, 1984.

71. Levy, D. E., et al.: Predicting outcome from hypoxic–ischemic coma. *JAMA* 253:1420–1426, 1985.

72. Lewy, R: *Preventive Primary Medicine*, Little, Brown & Company, Boston, 1980.

73. Macleod, J.: *Clinical Examination*, 5th ed., Churchill Livingstone, Edinburgh, 1979.

74. Matas, B. R.: The optic fundus and hypertension. *Med Clin North Am* 61:547–564, 1977.

75. Mayo Clinic and Mayo Foundation: *Clinical Examinations in Neurology*, 5th ed., W. B. Saunders Company, Philadelphia, 1981.

76. McAdam, L. P., et al.: Relapsing polychondritis. *Medicine* 55:193–215, 1976.

77. McCarty, D. J.: *Arthritis and Allied Conditions*, 10th ed., Lea and Febiger, Philadelphia, 1985.

78. McLoughlin, M. J., et al.: Abdominal bruits. *JAMA* 232:1238–1242, 1975.

79. Messerli, F. H., et al.: Osler's Maneuver and pseudohypertension. *N Engl J Med* 312:1548–1551, 1985.

80. Michiels, J. J., et al.: Erythromelalgia caused by platelet-mediated arteriolar inflammation and thrombosis in thrombocythemia. *Ann Intern Med* 102:466–471, 1985.

81. Millikan, C. H., et al.: A classification and outline of cerebrovascular diseases II. *Stroke* 6:565–616, 1975.

82. Mills, J. and Ho, M. T.: *Current Emergency Diagnosis and Treatment*, 2nd ed., Lange Medical Publications, Los Altos, 1985.

83. Morgan, W. L., Jr., and Engel, G. L.: *The Clinical Approach to the Patient*, W. B. Saunders Company, Philadelphia, 1969.

84. Murphy, R. L. H., et al.: Visual lung-sound characterization by time-expanded wave-form analysis. *N Engl J Med* 296:968–970, 1977.

85. Murphy, R. L. H. and Holford, S. K.: Lung sounds. *Basics of RD* (4):1–6, 1980.

86. Newell, F. W.: *Ophthalmology, Principles and Concepts*, 5th ed., C. V. Mosby Company, St. Louis, 1982.

87. O'Brien, E. and O'Malley, K.: *Essentials of Blood Pressure Measurement*, Churchill Livingstone, Edinburgh, 1981.

88. Paletta, F. X.: Dupuytren's contracture. *Am Fam Physician* 23:85–90, 1981.

89. Paton, D., et al: *Introduction to Ophthalmoscopy*, Upjohn Company, Kalamazoo, 1976.

90. Patz, A.: Retinal vascular diseases. *N Engl J Med* 298:1451–1454, 1978.

91. Perloff, J. K.: *Physical Examination of the Heart and Circulation*, W. B. Saunders Company, Philadelphia, 1982.

92. Petersdorf, R. G.: *Harrison's Principles of Internal Medicine*, 10th ed., McGraw–Hill Book Company, New York, 1983.

93. Plum, F. and Posner, J. B.: *The Diagnosis of Stupor and Coma*, 3rd ed., F. A. Davis Company, Philadelphia, 1980.

94. Polley, H. F. and Hunder, G. G.: *Rheumatologic Interviewing and Physical Examination of the Joints*, 2nd ed., W. B. Saunders Company, Philadelphia, 1978.

95. Prior, J. A., et al.: *Physical Diagnosis*, 6th ed., C. V. Mosby Company, St. Louis, 1981.

96. Reed, C. E.: The pathogenesis of asthma. *Med Clin North Am* 58:55–63, 1974.

97. Rodnan G. P., et al.: *Primer on the Rheumatic Diseases*, 8th ed., The Arthritis Foundation, New York, 1983.

98. Roederer, G. O., et al.: The natural history of carotid arterial disease in asymptomatic patients with cervical bruits. *Stroke* 15:605–613, 1984.

99. Rosenman, R. H., et al.: Relation of corneal arcus to cardiovascular risk factors and the incidence of coronary disease. *N Engl J Med* 291:1322–1324, 1974.

100. Ryan, R. E., et al.: *Synopsis of Ear, Nose, and Throat Diseases*, 3rd ed., C. V. Mosby Company, St. Louis, 1970.

101. Sandok, B. A., et al.: Carotid artery bruits. *Mayo Clin Proc* 57:227–230, 1982.

102. Shaver, J. A. and O'Toole, J. D.: The second heart sound: newer concepts. *Mod Concepts Cardiovasc Dis* XLVI:7–12, 1977.

103. Sherlock, S.: *Diseases of the Liver and Biliary System*, 6th ed., Blackwell Scientific Publications, Oxford, 1981.

104. Silen, W.: *Cope's Early Diagnosis of the Acute Abdomen*, 16th ed., W. B. Saunders Company, Philadelphia, 1983.

105. Slap, G. B., et al.: When to perform biopsies of enlarged peripheral lymph nodes in young patients. *JAMA* 252:1321–1326, 1984.

106. Smith, D. R.: *General Urology*, 11th ed., Lange Medical Publications, Los Altos, 1984.

107. Smith, N. D., et al.: Auscultation of the normally functioning prosthetic valve. *Ann Intern Med* 95:594–598, 1981.

108. Spittel, J. A.: *Clinical Medicine*, (2)18:3, Harper & Row Publishers, Philadelphia, 1985.

109. Spittel, J. A.: *Clinical Medicine*, (1)2:50, Harper & Row Publishers, Philadelphia, 1985.

110. Stein, J. H.: *Internal Medicine*, Little, Brown & Company, Boston, 1983.

111. Stein, P. D. and Sabbah, H. N.: Aortic origin of innocent murmurs. *Am J Cardiol* 39:665–671, 1977.

112. Stewart, W. D., et al.: *Dermatology*, 4th ed., C. V. Mosby Company, St. Louis, 1978.

113. Strub, R. L. and Black, F. W.: *The Mental Status Examination in Neurology*, F. A. Davis Company, Philadelphia, 1977.

114. Swash, M. and Mason, S.: *Hutchison's Clinical Methods*, 18th ed., Bailliere Tindall, London, 1984.

115. Tandberg, D. and Sklar, D.: Effect of tachypnea on the estimation of body temperature by an oral thermometer. *N Engl J Med* 308:945–946, 1983.

116. Todd, J. K.: Staphylococcal toxin syndromes. *Ann Rev Med* 36:337–347, 1985.

117. Turner, W. D. and Gold, R. G.: *Auscultation of the Heart*, 5th ed., Churchill Livingstone, Edinburgh, 1984.

118. Van Allen, M. W. and Rodnitzky, R. L.: *Pictorial Manual of Neurologic Tests*, 2nd ed., Year Book Medical Publishers, Chicago, 1981.

119. Vaughn, D. and Asbury, T.: *General Ophthalmology*, 10th ed., Lange Medical Publications, Los Altos, 1983.

120. Walker, H. K., et al.: *Clinical Methods*, 2nd ed., Butterworths, Boston, 1980.

121. Welch A.: *A Guide to the Use of Diagnostic Instruments in Eye, Ear, Nose, and Throat Examinations*, 1982.

122. Wilson, J. D. and Foster, D. W.: *Williams Textbook of Endocrinology*, 7th ed., W. B. Saunders Company, Philadelphia, 1985.

123. Wintrobe, M. M., et al.: *Clinical Hematology*, 8th ed., Lea and Febiger, Philadelphia, 1981.

124. Wyngaarden, J. B. and Smith, L. H., Jr.: *Cecil Textbook of Medicine*, 17th ed., W. B. Saunders Company, Philadelphia, 1985.

125. Zatouroff, M.: *Color Atlas of Physical Signs in General Medicine*, Year Book Medical Publishers, Chicago, 1976.

Index

E

U

V